the essential green you

easy ways to detox your diet, your body, and your life

volume three in the bestselling green this! series

deirdre imus

simon & schuster paperbacks

new york   london   toronto   sydney

Simon & Schuster Paperbacks
A Division of Simon & Schuster, Inc.
1230 Avenue of the Americas
New York, NY 10020

First Simon & Schuster trade paperback edition January 2009

For information about special discounts for bulk purchases, please contact
Simon & Schuster Special Sales at 1-800-456-6798 or business@simonandschuster.com

Designed by Davina Mock-Maniscalco

Manufactured in the United States of America

10   8   6   4   2   1   3   5   7   9

Library of Congress Cataloging-in-Publication Data

Imus, Deirdre.
The essential green you: easy ways to detox your diet,
your body, and your life / Deirdre Imus.
p. cm.—(Green this! ; v. 3)
Includes bibliographical references.
1. Environmental responsibility.   2. Environmentalism.   3. Green products.   I. Title.
GE195.7.I48 2008
640—dc22
2007050947
ISBN-13: 978-1-4165-4125-7
ISBN-10:   1-4165-4125-X

"If you think you're too small to have an impact, try sleeping in a room with a mosquito."

—African proverb

Acknowledgments

Thank you to my wonderful writer Virginia Sole-Smith. You are a pleasure to work with.

Amanda Murray, my incredible editor, I thank you.

Thank you Esther Newberg for your constant honesty and guidance.

David Rosenthal, thank you.

Thanks to all the experts that contributed to the valuable information in this book.

Many thanks to Bonnie Eskenazi, Jim Ronchi, LaRae Muse, Erin Idhe, and David Marks at the Deirdre Imus Environmental Center for Pediatric Oncology.

Thank you Wyatt and Don for being my green guinea pigs.

Contents

the essential
green you

Chapter 1

Take Charge of Your Health

Let me start by asking you a question: What prompted you to pick up this book?

Perhaps you've read the earlier books in my Green This! series. You've already begun to green your cleaning products and take important steps to protect your children's health from environmental toxins—and now you're ready to green your own life as well. If so, congratulations on your efforts so far, and on your decision to start the next chapter in your new, healthier life.

Or perhaps you're brand new to the Green Revolution. You've heard news advisories not to eat mercury-laden fish or read an article or two about toxins in your personal-care products, but you're not really sure what it all means. If so, welcome. You're in the right place to learn more.

Maybe you or your mom, dad, or dear friend has suffered from cancer, asthma, or another chronic illness—and you've wondered why the doctors that treat these conditions don't know more about what causes them. If so, you're not alone. I've wondered too, and I'm eager to share the answers I've found.

Whatever your reason for picking up this book, one thing's for sure: You're about to begin improving your life. Because although medical advances are allowing us to live longer today than we did in the past, we're also facing more threats to our health than ever before. The vast petrochemical and agricultural industries that have developed in the decades since World War II have created some one hundred thousand synthetic chemicals, 90 percent of which have never been assessed for safety. Most of these simply did not exist when we were kids, which means we have no idea what they might do to us, or to our own kids growing up today.

I know when most people think "chemicals," they think of funny colored test tubes in laboratories or big, steaming vats locked up in factories. But most of these chemicals are in products we use and foods we eat every day. Whether it's a box of tissues, a tube of eyeliner, a bottle of cold medicine, or a bag of microwave popcorn, all of these goods are mass-produced by large corporations focused on the bottom line—not our health.

Shockingly little is known about how all of the chemicals we're absorbing interact with one another and with our body chemistry. What we do know is that we're sick. The World Health Organization estimates that our environment (our air, water, food, homes, and the products we use) significantly affects more than 80 percent of major diseases. Asthma, Alzheimer's disease, autism, birth defects, cancer, endometriosis, infertility, multiple sclerosis, and Parkinson's disease are increasingly common, and scientists are collecting mounting evidence linking their incidence with environmental toxins. Consider these facts:

- An estimated 125 million Americans (43 percent of the population) have at least one chronic illness; 60 million of these folks have multiple chronic conditions. (Source: National Chronic Care Consortium)

- In 1950, health officials predicted that 25 percent of all Americans would eventually be diagnosed with cancer.

By 1997 that figure had risen to more than 40 percent. One in three women and one in two men will develop cancer during their lifetime. (Source: The Bay Area Working Group on the Precautionary Principle)

- In the 1940s, a woman's lifetime risk of developing breast cancer was one in twenty-two. Today it's one in seven—and rising. (Source: The Breast Cancer Fund)

- The number of men diagnosed with breast cancer has increased 25 percent in the past twenty-five years. (Source: The Breast Cancer Fund)

- The prevalence of asthma in our population is doubling every twenty years. (Source: The Bay Area Working Group on the Precautionary Principle)

- Exposures to hazardous chemicals in the workplace kill more than sixty thousand U.S. workers each year. There are more than eight hundred thousand new cases of occupational disease each year. The annual cost of workplace-related diseases in the United States is $25.8 billion, representing a substantial drain on the U.S. economy and on the lives of workers and their families. (Source: The Healthy Californians Biomonitoring Program)

Connecting the Dots

Though genetics and family history certainly play a role, the increasing rates of these diseases can be explained mainly by one common denominator: Our toxic planet.

"Only one in ten women who develop breast cancer do so because they inherited a defective gene from their parents," says Devra Lee Davis, PhD, MPH, director of the Center for Environmental Oncology at the University of Pittsburgh Cancer Institute. "That means that nine out of ten women who get the disease were born with healthy genes. Something happened to those genes over the course of a lifetime to give them breast cancer."

The same can be said for almost every chronic illness out there. It's time to recognize how complicated and interconnected our web of life really is. The toxins in our environment are working their way into our bodies, corrupting our healthy genes, cells, and organs, and making us sick. The Centers for Disease Control and Prevention (CDC) has detected 148 separate chemicals in the blood and urine of Americans of all ages and races. In 2006, researchers at the nonprofit Environmental Working Group (EWG) studied four mother-daughter pairs and found that each woman's blood or urine was contaminated with an average of thirty-five consumer product ingredients, including flame retardants, plasticizers, and stain-proof coatings.

Some chemicals, like phthalates, which make plastic flexible, can be excreted out of our bodies daily but are so ubiquitous in our environment that we reabsorb them daily too. Other toxins, like lead, can stay put in our bones for the rest of our lives. Though this chemical exposure poses the most health risks to children, the EWG researchers note that the mothers harbored an average of 1.5 to 5.2 times more pollution in their bodies than their daughters. This shows that even small doses of these chemicals can build up in our bodies over the course of years, posing long-term, persistent health threats.

So we know chemicals are accumulating in our bodies. But how do we know if they're responsible for our skyrocketing rates of disease? A 2007 evidence review led by scientists at the Silent Spring Institute, a nonprofit research organization dedicated to identifying the links between our environment and women's health, identified 216 chemicals that studies have demonstrated can cause breast cancer in lab animals and cell cultures. Of these, 73 are commonly found in consumer goods like cosmetics, dyes, and drugs or as pesticide residue on food; another 35 are airborne pollutants found in gasoline and smog. The scientists published their findings in *Cancer,* the journal of the American Cancer Society.

In December 2006, Philippe Grandjean, MD, an adjunct professor in the Department of Environmental Health at the Harvard School of Public Health published an evidence review in the medical journal *The Lancet* identifying 201 chemicals shown to be toxic to the neurological system. Once again, most of the list is common ingredients in food and consumer goods. About half are chemicals that factories produce at the rate of more than 1 million pounds per year. And this is just the tip of the hundred-thousand-chemical iceberg: "Perhaps as many as 25 percent of the chemicals [in use worldwide] can be expected to show neurotoxic properties," Dr. Grandjean writes.

Many companies that manufacture all these chemicals will tell you "the dose makes the poison," but in fact, two decades of research now show the inadequacy of that belief. Timing, duration, and pattern of exposure are at least as important as the dose, so low-dose exposure to chemicals that are ubiquitous in our environment can cause permanent damage if it continues over a lifetime, or even just at the most vulnerable stages of our lives. We need to take a good, hard look at the chemicals we're using every day. Alternatives are out there and should be used.

A Time for Precaution, Not Panic

I know I've thrown a lot of scary facts and figures at you in just a few short pages, and you're probably feeling as frustrated as I did when I first began to learn about these threats. It's easy to get paralyzed by all this information—I often hear people say, "Oh well, we're all going to die anyway." But I'm not telling you these facts to make you panic or to resign you to your fate. I'm doing it to encourage you to join me in making easy, positive changes to reduce the number of toxic exposures in your life. Throughout this book I'll be giving you plenty of tips and ideas about what you can do to help. Just take it one step at a time. Focus on changing one thing in your life and making that stick, then worry about the next thing on the list. Every seemingly simple, fundamental change you make will do so much good for your health.

Most of the changes I advocate are based on what environmentalists call the "precautionary principle." In 1998, a coalition of scientists, philosophers, lawyers, and environmental activists defined the principle in a wingspread consensus statement. It goes something like this: "When an activity raises threats of harm to human health or the environment, precautionary measures should be taken even if some cause and effect relationships are not fully established scientifically. In this context the proponent of an activity, rather than the public, should bear the burden of proof. The process of applying the Precautionary Principle must be open, informed and democratic and must include potentially affected parties. It must also involve an examination of the full range of alternatives, including no action."

Or, as I like to say, "Better safe than sorry." In our complex world, scientists cannot always predict what impact toxic exposures will have on our health. We need to recognize the limits of our scientific knowledge and be willing to say "I don't know," even if it means we have to make changes to protect against a potential, but not yet proven, risk.

Industry hates the precautionary principle, because it puts the burden of proof on them and limits what they are allowed to make and sell until they can show that it's safe. But this makes it a cost-effective and caring strategy for you—it's always better, and more affordable, to prevent disease and pollution before they happen than to try to cure or clean up after the fact.

All you have to do to apply the precautionary principle to your life is pay attention and ask questions. Too often we walk through the aisles of our supermarkets and drugstores as if we're in a coma, never even looking at what we buy. The general consensus is that if it's on store shelves, it must be safe. But in fact, nothing could be further from the truth. Need proof? Remember that cigarettes are on those store shelves too.

As you start questioning and becoming more conscious of the products and foods you buy, you'll realize that the process can be never-ending. Our lifestyles have changed. The world is a busier, noisier, more industrialized, and more toxic place. But we can't compromise our health or the health of our children just because our schedules are fuller.

This book is here to help. I'll guide you through everything you put on or in your body (food, personal-care products, clothes, medications) and help you find easy ways to reduce your overall intake of toxins, whether they come in a jar of face cream or a bottle of salad dressing. Look out for my Eco Shopping List at the end of each chapter, where I'll suggest products and brands you can trust and tell you where to find them. And be sure to read the A Greener You sections, where you can find stories and tips from readers like you who have already taken small steps toward greening their lives. In the appendix you'll find a collection of my favorite recipes courtesy of Arlena Teitelbaum, the wonderful chef at the Imus Ranch.

As consumers, you have so much more power than you realize. It's time to ask what we're being exposed to every time we eat, shower, or get dressed—and why. We may not be able to change the world, but we can change the way we think about our health. Each one of us has tremendous potential to make a difference.

Chapter 2

Eating Green

I'm starting this book with a discussion of food for a simple reason that you've heard thousands of times: We are what we eat. In fact, if you're only going to read one chapter in this whole book, this is the one to read. In my opinion (and the opinion of many nutritionists and scientists), adopting a plant-based diet is the single most important thing you can do to improve your health.

It's no secret that Americans are fatter and unhealthier than we've ever been before, or that our $1 billion food industry has played a significant role in the decline of our health. Nevertheless, we are "a notably unhealthy people obsessed by the idea of eating healthily," as environmental journalist Michael Pollan writes in his groundbreaking book *The Omnivore's Dilemma*—and we're more confused about how to eat healthily than ever before.

It's time to take a closer look at every aspect of this industry and its impact on our lives. But this is not as easy as it sounds. For me it's been a long journey that began in high school, when I decided to stop eating meat and dairy to improve my performance as a runner. Part of it was teenage rebellion—I remember refusing to eat turkey and butter-soaked mashed potatoes at Thanksgiving. I ruined almost every holiday for my relatives because I was such a nightmare! But really I was just trying to figure out how to have a healthier relationship with food. I refused to go on autopilot and eat just anything put in front of me, even though that's the way my family ate and what most of us were brought up to do.

As I went on to college, I made every effort to learn about how meat and dairy foods impact our health. Much of the information I'm going to share with you in these next few chapters comes from the writers, scientists, and activists whose pioneering work helped shape my own perspective and who, in my mind, are the real heroes of our clean food revolution. Consider these next few chapters your crash course in Eating Green 101. If you want to learn more about any of the issues I introduce, I recommend the following books:

- *Diet for a New America* by John Robbins. Robbins grew up heir to the Baskin-Robbins ice cream fortune but walked away from the family business in order to pursue "a dream of a society that is truly healthy, practicing a wise and compassionate stewardship of a balanced ecosystem." Published in 1987, this was the first book to connect the dots between our health, the health of the planet, and the importance of a plant-based diet. The book was so revolutionary at that time that Robbins reported beef consumption in the United States dropped nearly 20 percent in the five years following its publication. Robbins went on to found the influential vegan advocacy group EarthSave International.

- *The China Study* by T. Colin Campbell, PhD, and Thomas M. Campbell II. This book, published in 2005, reports the findings of the most comprehensive nutrition study every conducted. Dr. Campbell's team of researchers measured 367 diet, lifestyle, and disease-related variables among 6,500 Chinese adults, generating more than eight thousand statistically significant associations. His conclusions, some of which I'll discuss in this chapter, will shock and surprise you.

- *The Omnivore's Dilemma* by Michael Pollan. In this book Pollan follows four different food chains—industrial, organic, industrial organic, and hunter-gatherer—from their origins as seeds in soil all the way to your table. His intrepid reporting uncovers many frightening and important facts about the way we produce food today.

A Story of Three Farms

My evolution as a green eater hasn't stopped. I'm always learning more about how food can better sustain us. And the more I learn, the more committed I am to my vegan, all-organic lifestyle. But I'm not here to convince you to eat every meal exactly the way I do. There are many perfectly valid ways of eating green, and some of the most eco-conscious diners I know are still putting animal products on their plates. We don't necessarily agree on everything—in fact, we can have some pretty spirited debates! But what we all have in common is the simple knowledge that good health comes from good food—and good food comes from good soil.

You're probably thinking that's oversimplifying it a bit. And how does a slice of ham or a chicken drumstick come from soil? Well, remember: We are what we eat. And that means we are what they ate, too. Cows are vegetarians by nature, which means they eat grasses and grains that are grown in—you guessed it—soil. The quality of soil and the methods a farmer uses to reap food from it, whether he's harvesting tomatoes for our salads or growing grass to feed his dairy cow, are the first and most crucial steps in determining the quality of the food that ends up on our plate.

This is a lesson I've learned from three very different farms. One is our own Imus Cattle Ranch for Kids with Cancer in Ribera, New Mexico. We raise Texas Longhorn cattle, sheep, buffalo, chickens, goats, and donkeys on nearly four thousand acres and grow a wide range of fruits, vegetables, and herbs, most in our state-of-the-art greenhouse. The second is the Stone Barns Center for Food and Agriculture in New York's Hudson River valley, where farmers raise Berkshire hogs, sheep, and poultry on fifteen acres and grow an enormous variety of vegetables in their greenhouse and gardens. The third is Polyface Farm in Swoope, Virginia, which Pollan profiles in *The Omnivore's Dilemma* and which inspired many of the techniques used at Stone Barns. Joel Salatin, who raises chickens, turkeys, cattle, rabbits, and pigs, plus tomatoes, sweet corn, and berries on his 100 acres of pasture and 450 acres of forest, calls himself a "grass farmer" and considers soil to be "xthe earth's stomach" because, as Pollan explains, "a healthy soil digests the dead to nourish the living." None of our farms would grow a thing if we didn't first build the right kind of soil.

Each of these farms are practicing a kind of agriculture that is now termed "beyond organic" or sometimes "biodynamic." We've created living, breathing, and almost entirely self-sustaining ecosystems. Pigs forage in forests, fertilizing the soil with their manure. Sheep and cattle graze pasture, followed by chickens, who eat the leftover grasses, then peck apart their manure to rejuvenate the soil. And vegetables are rotated seasonally with cover crops to recycle nutrients back into the soil that feeds them. None of these farms use chemicals of any kind— no herbicides, insecticides, pesticides, growth hormones, or antibiotics. We don't need them because these ecosystems stay healthy all on their own, thanks to the incredible soil digesting and nourishing it all. And when these farms stay healthy, the food they produce is the healthiest you could ever hope to eat.

Unfortunately, most of the industrial farms raising our food aren't designed on this self-sustaining, beyond-organic model, and we're paying the price: The Center for Science in the Public Interest (CSPI) reports that American croplands lose 2 billion tons of topsoil to erosion annually. Because there is such a huge demand for the grains that feed commercially raised livestock, many large-scale farmers now do what's called "monocropping," where they raise single crops over huge areas. Planting and replanting the same one or two crops in the same spots season after season causes erosion and depletes the remaining soil of its nutrients.

A Clean Food Revolution

As a result of the healthy practices of farms like Stone Barns and Polyface, the food they produce is of the highest quality, conferring many health benefits not found in conventionally raised beef, pork, lamb, and poultry. But as I'll show you in the pages to come, that doesn't mean animal products in general are the best choices for our health. A huge body of scientific evidence from the China Study and many other sources demonstrates that our Western diet, which relies so heavily on animal protein and fat (as well as refined carbohydrates) is killing us. Consider these facts (all from research by EarthSave International and CSPI):

- Vegetarians have a 28 percent lower death rate from heart disease than meat eaters.

- The saturated fat and cholesterol in beef, pork, dairy foods, poultry, and eggs cause about 63,000 fatal heart attacks each year.

- Women who eat red meat once a day have a 250-percent increased chance of getting colon cancer compared with women who eat it less than once a month.

- More than 60 percent of Americans are overweight, with at least 30 percent considered obese, compared with an obesity rate of 6 percent among vegetarians and 2 percent among vegans.

- As many as 75 percent of women who eat fish more than twice a week possess blood levels of mercury, a known neurotoxin, that are seven times higher than women who don't eat fish at all.

- The death rate of breast cancer among American women is 350 percent higher than the rate among Japanese women and nearly 500 percent the rate of Chinese women. (People in both China and Japan consume a diet high in fruits and vegetables and low in animal products.)

"Even relatively small intakes of animal-based foods could encourage biological processes that, over a lifetime, give rise to higher risks for a wide variety of cancers, cardiovascular diseases and diabetes," writes Dr. T. Colin Campbell. There's no question about it. We are slowly poisoning ourselves with our meat-based diets.

For these reasons and many more, eating vegan as well as "beyond organic" makes the most sense to me. But this is a personal choice everyone should make for him- or herself. And it's not one you should make overnight! After all, researchers at Cornell University's Food and Brand Lab report that we're faced with more than two hundred food-related decisions every day—you can't green every single one of them in one fell swoop. It took me years of reading, learning, and talking to scientists, nutritionists, farmers, and chefs to get here. But I'm ready to educate you on the key issues, so you can start to incorporate a little more knowledge and awareness into each of your food choices.

Start small. Green one meal a day, or even just one food in your fridge. Stick with it until that habit becomes second nature, and then add on. Whatever you decide to eat, remember that this process is not about depriving you of delicious meals or limiting the variety of wonderful foods you can eat. "Most of us just eat without thinking about flavor or where our food comes from," says Deborah Madison, author of the award-winning *Local Flavors: Cooking and Eating from America's Farmers' Markets, Vegetarian Cooking for Everyone,* and eight other wonderful cookbooks that have helped countless readers, myself included, embrace a healthy and delicious plant-based diet. "All of these changes that help you eat well and take better care of yourself are also about moving towards a better quality life."

Activist Spotlight
Center for Science in the Public Interest

If you ever look at a food label to figure out if it's good or bad for you, thank the Center for Science in the Public Interest. This nonprofit health advocacy organization led the campaign that resulted in Congress passing the Nutrition Labeling and Education Act of 1990 requiring food manufacturers to put nutrition information and ingredient lists on their goods. More recently, CSPI worked to ensure the Food and Drug Administration's ban on trans fat (more on both of these issues in chapter 4). But their most important work, to my mind, has been their Eating Green campaign. "It struck me that a lot of the work we were doing was piecemeal," explains Michael Jacobson, PhD, one of CSPI's cofounders and now its executive director. "We were telling people to avoid this or look for that, but the big picture is that the healthiest way to eat is to load up on fruits, vegetables, and whole grains."

Greening your own diet can have a big impact. Swap one serving of beef, one egg, and one serving of cheese with a mix of fruits, veggies, beans, and whole grains each day and you will

- Increase your daily consumption of dietary fiber by 16 grams (more than half the recommended intake)
- Reduce your daily intake of fat by 22 grams (one-third the recommended daily limit) and saturated fat by 12 grams (more than half the recommended limit)
- Spare the need for 1.8 acres of cropland and 40 pounds of fertilizer
- Prevent 11,400 pounds of animal manure from being dumped into the environment each year, reducing air and water pollution

You can calculate the environmental and health impacts of your own diet and learn more about all these issues by visiting www.cspinet.org and www.eatinggreen.org.

Beef and Dairy

As I've already shown, an animal-based diet is at the root of why we're all so sick. And there's no question that red meat and dairy foods are some of the worst health offenders. It all starts with how these foods are raised. EarthSave reports that more than 80 percent of the cattle raised in the United States are confined to crowded feedlots—called concentrated animal feeding operations (CAFOs)—where they spend the majority of their lives getting little to no exercise or access to pasture. The goal of a CAFO is to get animals as fat as possible as quickly as possible, so cattle are fed huge quantities of high-calorie grains (usually corn), even though their stomachs have evolved to eat only grass. The unnatural diet causes a range of health problems, which CAFOs treat by dosing their cattle with huge amounts of antibiotics. But this poses risks as well. "Growing scientific evidence shows that the use of similar antibiotics in both human medicine and food animal production can erode the effectiveness of drugs vital for use in human medicine," reports Keep Antibiotics Working, a nonprofit alliance of public health advocacy groups. For more details on antibiotic resistance, see chapter 8.

Dairy cattle are raised in similarly confined conditions and fed daily doses of recombinant bovine growth hormone or bovine soma-totropin (known as rBGH or rBST), synthetic estrogen-mimicking hor-mones that increase the cows' milk production but also cause severe calcium deficiencies and frequent udder infections called mastitis. To treat these side effects, the cows are also dosed with daily antibiotics, and some studies show that trace amounts of the medicine can end up in conventional milk. To maintain production, year-round dairy cattle are kept pregnant or lactating three hundred days per year, and studies have also shown that the increased estrogen levels that result find their way into commercially produced milk.

These huge CAFOs and industrial dairy farms take an enormous toll on our environment as well. An average feedlot with ten thousand cows produces five hundred-thousand pounds of manure per day, reports EarthSave. "Livestock waste is responsible for 18 percent of greenhouse gas emissions, outranking cars," says Dr. Jacobson, also noting that 14 trillion gallons of water are needed to produce feed for all our livestock each year, with eighteen thousand gallons of rain and irrigation water needed to produce just one pound of beef.

And all of this comes back to haunt our health, whether in the form of toxic drinking water and filthy air or in the cheeseburgers we eat. As much as 95 percent of our exposure to dioxins (a class of highly toxic chemicals linked to cancer, birth defects, decreased fertility, learning disabilities, immune system suppression, lung problems, skin disorders, and more) comes from meat and dairy consumption. Ground beef, rib steak, and blue cheese contain the highest levels of dioxin, according to the Environmental Protection Agency's Dioxin Reassessment Summary, because of their high fat content. Dioxin, which is released into our environment through industrial processes like chlorine bleaching, accumulates in animal fat.

Countries that consume the most dairy have the highest rates of prostate, testicular, breast, ovarian, and uterine cancer. At least fifty studies from the past three decades link consumption of milk from cows treated with rBGH [and rBST] to increased risk for cancer, says Samuel Epstein, MD, founder of the Cancer Prevention Coalition, noting that both the European Union and Canada have banned the use of the growth hormone. rBGH milk can contain up to ten times the usual amount of a naturally occurring substance called insulin-like growth factor (IGF), which we then absorb across our intestinal walls into our bloodstreams and then into our bodies. Although the FDA says it's safe, some studies show that elevated levels of IGF-1 may promote transformation of normal breast cells to breast cancers; Dr. Epstein and other scientists suspect it plays a role in the development of other cancers and an increase in twin rates as well.

Harvard School of Public Health researchers agree that "there may be potential harm in consuming high amounts of dairy," as preliminary studies suggest that consuming high levels of galactose (a sugar released by the digestion of lactose in milk) may damage the ovaries and lead to ovarian cancer. And at least nine studies show a link between milk consumption and prostate cancer. In one Harvard study of male health professionals, those who drank two or more glasses of milk daily were almost twice as likely to develop advanced prostate cancer as those who didn't drink milk at all.

There is also the important point that most of us just aren't designed to digest milk. Evolutionary scientists calculate that it's only in the past ten thousand years that we've been able to safely digest dairy as adults, and even today, 90 percent of Asians, 70 percent of blacks and native Americans, 50 percent of Hispanics, and 15 percent of people of northern European descent are lactose intolerant, according to the Harvard School of Public Health.

Of course, many experts claim we need to drink milk to build strong, healthy bones, but the data on this isn't nearly as solid as most of us think. The Harvard Nurses' Health Study on 78,000 women found no evidence at all that higher intakes of milk reduced osteoporosis or the incidence of bone fractures. In fact, the study found that the relative risk of hip fracture for women who drink two glasses of milk per day was 1.45 times higher than those who drink one glass or less per week.

And don't forget that both milk and beef can be potent sources of artery-clogging saturated fat. Two 12-ounce glasses of whole milk contain as much saturated fat as a Big Mac and fries, notes EarthSave, while even one glass of 2-percent milk has as much as three strips of bacon. That corn-fed diet used on factory farms is certainly to blame— meat from a typical grain-fed steer is 100 percent fattier than meat from a grass-fed steer.

Processed meats like hot dogs (along with bacon and smoked hams) are some of the worst meat you can eat, because they not only contain high levels of dioxins and saturated fat, most are also treated with preservatives called nitrates. During the cooking process and possibly also in the human stomach, nitrates combine with other compounds to form N-nitroso compounds. These are known carcinogens associated with cancer of the oral cavity, urinary bladder, esophagus, stomach, and brain. A 1994 study found that children eating more than twelve hot dogs per month have nine times the normal risk of developing childhood leukemia, says Dr. Epstein. A strong risk also existed for children whose father's intake of hot dogs was twelve or more per month, according to a seven year study of Los Angeles County children from birth to age ten, published in 1987. Denver researchers found that children born to mothers who consumed hot dogs one or more times per week during pregnancy had approximately double the risk of developing brain tumors.

Shop Smarter

If you do decide to consume beef and dairy, here are some ways to maximize their health benefits and minimize their risks.

Best Bets

- **Grass-Fed or Pasture-Raised.** This means the cow was raised grazing pasture (its natural diet) instead of eating grain. "Grass-fed beef is one of the most sustainable and healthy products you can buy," says Pollan. In addition to being lower in saturated fat, grass-fed beef contains about five times as much omega-3 fatty acids as grain-fed beef. These essential fatty acids have many health benefits, including potentially reducing your risk for heart attack and stroke. "A growing body of research suggests that many of the health problems associated with eating beef are really problems with corn-fed beef," Pollan writes in *The Omnivore's Dilemma*. "Modern-day hunter-gatherers who subsist on wild meat don't have our rates of heart disease."

- **Certified Organic.** This label can only be used on meat and dairy foods that were produced in facilities that meet the United States Department of Agriculture's organic standards. They must be fed only organically grown feed (grain or grass that is not genetically modified and is grown without synthetic fertilizers, chemicals, or sewage sludge, without any animal byproducts mixed in) and cannot be treated with hormones or antibiotics. They must have access to the outdoors and pasture, though they do not need to be on an exclusively grass diet.

- **Certified Humane Raised and Handled.** This label is bestowed by the American Humane Society on animal products that meet their criteria for animal welfare. In the case of beef and dairy, it ensures that the cows were raised on pasture, allowed to engage in their natural grazing behaviors, and not fed antibiotics or growth hormones. For more info, visit www.certifiedhumane.org.

- **Fat Free.** Skim milk and cheese contain virtually no dioxins (since they accumulate in fat) and they're also lower in the heart-damaging saturated fat.

- **Nitrite Free.** Hot dogs with this label won't be as red as those treated with nitrites, but they are "perfectly safe and healthy," according to Dr. Epstein.

Better than Nothing

- **rBGH free and rBST free.** You'll find this label on many brands of nonorganic milk, and it should mean the cows weren't treated with growth hormones. But this label isn't regulated by the government, so double-check with the manufacturer that they have been certified to make this claim by Rural Vermont, a nonprofit farmer advocacy organization. For a list of approved dairies see my Eco Shopping List on page 37.

- **Food Alliance Approved.** Any meat with this label is from a ranch that has been verified by third-party inspectors to guarantee that it attempts to preserve soil and water quality and provides cattle with fresh air, pasture, and comfortable living quarters. FAA cows aren't allowed to be treated with hormones or unnecessary antibiotics. For more info visit www.foodalliance.org; you'll find these meats at farmers' markets, natural food stores in the Northwest and Midwest, and online.

- **Lamb and Goat.** Opt for these if you can't find organic or rBGH-free beef and dairy. Growth hormones cannot be used on these animals.

Pork

We raise between 60 and 90 million pigs per year on CAFOs, which pile up their waste in toxic manure lagoons. These lagoons release toxic chemicals into our air and often pollute our water (the Sierra Club reports that hog, chicken, and cattle waste combined has polluted 35,000 miles of rivers in twenty-two states and contaminated groundwater in seventeen states). Levels of hydrogen sulfide from the manure lagoon at one hog CAFO in Minnesota exceed the safe level for human health 271 times in two years, says the EPA. In one study it was found in the air at unsafe levels almost five miles from the source. In Indiana, the toxins released by hog waste were linked to six miscarriages in women living near a hog factory. And spills from these manure lagoons have also killed billions of fish and contaminated waterways across the country. In fact, animal waste flowing from the Mississippi River has helped to create a dead zone in the Gulf of Mexico that has grown to the size of New Jersey.

In addition to the toxicity of pig farming, don't forget the health risks of pig meat itself. Though not quite as fatty as grain-fed beef, pork contains plenty of saturated fat and thus is also a source of dioxin exposure. Processed pork, such as breakfast sausage, ham, and bacon is a major source of nitrites and also very high in sodium. A study by the Center for Science in the Public Interest found that a three-link serving of Johnsonville Original breakfast sausage has 610 milligrams of sodium—more than a quarter of what's safe for us to consume per day.

Shop Smarter

If you decide to consume pork, here's what you should look for at the meat counter.

Best Bets

- **Certified Organic or Certified Humane Raised and Handled.** See "Beef and Dairy" for more info.

- **Raised on Small Family Farms.** This label should mean that pigs have plenty of access to the outdoors so they can indulge their natural foraging behavior, as they do at Stone Barns. Look for it at farmers' markets or natural grocery stores (be sure to ask your grocer where the product is sourced, as there's no legal definition for this label).

- **Nitrite Free.** See "Beef and Dairy" for more info.

Poultry and Eggs

Chickens need access to the outdoors so they can forage for the grasses, grain seeds, insects, and minerals that make up their natural diet. But 99 percent of laying hens in CAFOs live their entire lives in wire cages, where they're fed a mash of refined grains (corn and sorghum), cottonseed meal, or soybean oil meal. Protein and fat is added to their diet in the form of bone, meat, poultry feathers, pet litter, and other animal byproducts from poultry, beef, and swine.

The tight quarters make them more prone to a variety of health problems that farmers treat by giving the birds a steady diet of antibiotics. According to a recent report from the Union of Concerned Scientists, 10.5 million pounds of antibiotics are administered in poultry production each year, versus 3 million pounds for human medicine. Broiler chickens (killed for their meat) are also pumped full of antibiotics and other growth-promoting drugs so that they grow six times more quickly than normal, ending up so top-heavy they are barely able to move.

The result: anemic, unhealthy meat "enhanced" by poultry producers with as much as 15 percent saltwater to improve flavor. The Center for Science in the Public Interest reported that that this so-called natural chicken contains up to five times as much sodium as regular chicken.

Conventionally raised eggs also suffer on the nutrition front, containing far less omega-3 fatty acids, beta-carotene, and vitamin E than organic, sustainably farmed eggs. And the government reports that 2.3 million eggs each year are contaminated with *Salmonella* bacteria.

Shop Smarter

Best Bets

- **Certified Organic or Certified Humane Raised and Handled.** See "Beef and Dairy" for details.

- **Pasture Raised.** Guarantees that the chickens were raised outdoors and able to engage in their natural pecking behavior. It's hard to find this label at supermarkets; your best bet is to buy eggs and chicken from a local farmers' market where you can ask the farmer how she raises her birds.

- **Biodynamic.** This is a verified label (also found on some beef and pork) meaning the hens were raised outdoors (weather permitting), were not fed any growth-promoting drugs or antibiotics, were not subject to pesticide exposure, were vegetarian fed with biodynamic feed, were not debeaked, and were not force-molted (a practice where older laying hens are starved of food and light for several days until they lay their last round of eggs).

- **Free Farmed.** This label is verified by Farm Animal Services, a branch of the American Humane Association. Their standards include access to clean water, food, and the outdoors, prohibition of forced molting, elimination of antibiotics used for growth promotion, and hygienic waste-management practices.

Better than Nothing

- **Cage Free.** This label means the chickens were spared the brutality of life in wire cages, but because this term is not officially defined by the U.S. Department of Agriculture, it doesn't tell you whether the birds were raised outdoors on pasture, in a barn with access to the outdoors, or lived their entire lives inside in overcrowded conditions, just minus the literal cage. If you see this label, ask your grocer or the farmer (if you're at your farmers' market) for more info.

Don't Fall For

- **Free Range.** The USDA allows this label on any chicken that is given "some access to the outdoors each day," but it doesn't guarantee that chickens are given this access for any specific amount of time nor does it ensure that they actually go outside during that time or that they live in hygienic cage-free environments the rest of the time.

- **Antibiotic Free.** This term should mean the hens weren't given any antibiotics, but it's only verified if the poultry is also labeled as "Certified Organic," according to a report by Consumers Union.

- **No Additives.** The USDA only requires that this mean no additives were applied to the eggs themselves. It doesn't have anything to do with what the chickens were fed, nor does it ensure that no antibiotics or pesticides were used to treat the birds.

- **No Chemicals Added.** Again, this label only means no chemicals were added to the eggs themselves, says Consumers Union, which isn't very meaningful considering that farmers have no reason to inject chemicals into fragile eggshells. It's not verified by an independent third party and has nothing to do with the feed, antibiotics, or other drugs given to chickens while they were laying.

- **No Hormones Administered.** This is a misleading claim often printed on chickens and eggs, even though a federal law bans the use of hormones in poultry (though not in cattle or pigs). The law does not prevent chicken farmers from feeding their flock large doses of growth-promoting antibiotics and other drugs that may act like hormones in the body.

Fish

Fish are often touted as a kind of wonder food—if you believe everything you see on TV, salmon can do everything from curing attention deficit disorder to erasing wrinkles! In fact, while fish are good sources of lean protein and essential fatty acids, too much of the wrong kinds can put you at risk for mercury poisoning and other chemical exposures. Mercury is a heavy metal that pollutes our air and water thanks to coal-burning power plants and can impair brain development in a fetus or young child. It also plays a role in the development of cardiovascular disease, according to a June 2007 study published in the *International Journal of Toxicology*. Because it is fat soluble, mercury accumulates in fish (especially large, predatory species) and is easily absorbed into our bodies when we eat them. As a result, one in five women nationwide has mercury levels higher than the EPA limit, according to a 2006 Sierra Club report that analyzed hair samples from 6,600 volunteers from all fifty states.

In 1985, 95 percent of the fish we ate were caught in the wild, reports EarthSave. By 2000, one-third of the fish we ate came from fish farms (including 40 percent of all salmon), and that number is climbing. These farms are rife with disease and pollution, as mercury and other chemicals become even more concentrated in the close quarters. Farmed salmon contains eleven times more dioxin than wild-caught salmon and nearly eight times the level of polychlorinated biphenyls (also called PCBs, a class of industrial chemicals banned in 1977 that still persist in the environment), according to a 2004 study in the journal *Science*.

Farmed fish are also lower in omega-3 fatty acids, which wild fish manufacture from eating algae. Like cattle, pigs, and chicken, farmed fish are fed mostly grain mixed with ground-up smaller fish, and as a result, "the omega-3 levels of farmed salmon fall well below those of wild fish," writes Pollan. "Conventional nutritional wisdom holds that salmon is automatically better for us than beef, but that judgment assumes the beef has been grain fed and the salmon krill fed; if the steer is fattened on grass and the salmon on grain, we might actually be better off eating the beef."

Shop Smarter

If you do decide to eat fish, the Institute for Agriculture and Trade Policy (or IATP, a research and advocacy group that promotes the preservation of our ecosystems and family farms) recommends choosing small fish that are low on the food chain, as they accumulate fewer toxins than big fish. Stick to small portion sizes (a 3-ounce serving is about the size of a deck of cards), trim excess fat, and broil, bake, or grill fish so the fat (which contains most of the PCBs and dioxins) drips away. Deep-frying and panfrying will concentrate chemicals.

Here's a guide to eating safer fish that are also fished with minimal destruction to the environment, culled from the experts at the *Green Guide,* IATP, and the Environmental Working Group:

Avoid

Stay away from these fish, especially if you're pregnant; these species are overfished, farmed destructively, and/or high in toxins.

- Arctic char (freshwater)
- Bass, including Chilean and white sea bass (also called Gulf corvina)
- Catfish (wild)
- Caviar (Russian and Iranian)
- Cod (Atlantic)
- Conch, queen
- Crab, king (imported)
- Croaker (Pacific)
- Flounder (Atlantic)
- Grenadier
- Groupers
- Haddock (trawl caught)
- Hake, white
- Halibut (Atlantic)
- Lobster (Caribbean, and all imported spiny except Australian)
- Mackerel, king and Spanish
- Mahi-mahi (imported long line)
- Marlin
- Monkfish
- Octopus (imported, troll caught)
- Opah
- Orange roughy

- Oysters (eastern and Gulf Coast)
- Pike
- Pompano (Florida)
- Rockfish (including trawl caught and Pacific red snapper)
- Salmon (farmed)
- Sea scallops (United States and mid-Atlantic)
- Sea turtles
- Shark
- Shrimp (imported)
- Skate
- Snapper (red or imported)
- Sole (Atlantic)
- Sturgeon (wild caught)
- Swordfish
- Tilapia (China, Taiwan farmed)
- Tilefish
- Totoaba
- Tuna (albacore, bigeye, bluefin, yellowfin)
- Turbot (greenland halibut)
- Yellow Perch

Safe to Eat Once a Month

These species represent recovering populations and/or only contain moderate levels of mercury.

- Bass, striped (farmed)
- Bluefish
- Calamari
- Clams (caught)
- Cod (Pacific)
- Crab (including Gulf Coast blue, Alaskan king, Hawaiian and Australian Kona, Alaskan snow)
- Flounder (Pacific)
- Haddock (hook and line)
- Hake (silver, red, and offshore/wild caught)
- Halibut (Pacific and wild caught)
- Jacksmelt
- Lobster (Maine)
- Mackerel, Spanish (Atlantic)
- Mahi-mahi (troll-caught)
- Mussels, Blue
- Octopus (Hawaiian, Gulf of California, wild caught)
- Pomfret, big-scale
- Prawn (American, wild caught)
- Sablefish/black cod
- Salmon (California, Washington, or wild caught)
- Sand dabs
- Scup/porgy

- Shrimp (American, Atlantic, Gulf of Mexico; farmed or trawl-caught and wild-caught Canadian northern)

- Sole (Pacific)

- Squid, jumbo (Gulf of California)

- Tilapia (Central America farmed)

- Trevally

- Tuna (canned light)

- Tuna (troll-caught Pacific albacore)

Safe to Eat

These seafood products are low in mercury and not overfished or farmed destructively.

- Abalone (farmed)

- Anchovies

- Artic char (farmed)

- Barramundi (American farmed)

- Catfish (American farmed)

- Caviar (American or French farmed)

- Clams, soft-shelled or steamer (farmed)

- Crab (trap-caught American Dungeness, Alaskan wild-caught imitation, Canadian snow, Florida stone)

- Crawfish (American farmed)

- Croaker (Atlantic)

- Cuttlefish
- Herring
- Hoki
- Lobster, spiny or rock (American, Australian, Baja west coast)
- Mackerel, Atlantic (purse-seine caught)
- Mussels (American farmed)
- Oysters (Pacific farmed)
- Pollock (Alaskan wild caught)
- Prawn (British Columbian wild caught)
- Salmon (Alaskan wild caught)
- Sardines
- Scad, big-eye and mackerel (Hawaiian)
- Scallops, bay (American farmed)
- Shrimp, pink or wild-caught
- Squid, longfin (American, Atlantic)
- Sturgeon (farmed)
- Tilapia (American farmed)
- Trout, rainbow (American farmed)

Eco Shopping List

Choosing a plant-based diet can seem like hard work at first, and you can expect to get plenty of questions and odd looks from folks, especially when you're trying to navigate a restaurant menu. I hate preachy vegans and don't think you should give lectures at the dinner table, but I do get annoyed when people give us a hard time about eating healthy, because it's a symptom of what's wrong with our food system. In a perfect world, it would be the folks who want to eat unhealthy hormone- and pesticide-laden food who would seem strange to the rest of us.

I also hear a lot of people complain about cost. No question about it, grass-fed beef costs significantly more than conventional supermarket beef, organic milk can often be double the price of conventional, and so on. Of course you'll save plenty of money if you stop eating these foods altogether! Even if you just reduce your consumption, you may find the overall savings offset your sticker shock. But until a larger market is created for these foods, you have to view the increased cost as a way to vote with your dollars. The more we shop this way, the more we'll save in the long run because society will not bear the cost of the conventional food supply's environmental pollution and health consequences. I think that's worth making sustainable, healthy food a priority, even if you have to cut back spending in other areas of your life. "We Americans spend only a fraction of our disposable income feeding ourselves—about a tenth, down from a fifth in the 1950s," writes Pollan. "This suggests that there are many of us who could afford to spend more on food *if we chose to*. After all, it isn't only the elite who in recent years have found an extra fifty or one hundred dollars each month to spend on cell phones."

I'm not asking you to double your food budget or give up meat and dairy overnight. But consider make small changes in your diet and I suspect you'll soon find the benefits are well worth the effort.

Vegan Pantry Staples

If you decide to go ahead and clear the meat and dairy foods out of your fridge, you might be wondering what should take their place. I keep these staples on hand at all times. You should be able to find all of these at your local supermarket or health food store. I've included brand names where applicable. Choose organic whenever possible!

Nuts and Seeds

I buy these from the bulk bins at my local health food store.

- Raw pumpkin seeds (or tossed in safflower oil and sea salt, then baked for twenty minutes for a crunchy, tasty snack)
- Sunflower seeds
- Ground flaxseed
- Raw almonds
- Tamari almonds
- Raw filberts
- Raw cashews
- Raw walnuts
- Raw pecans

Fruit

Also found in bulk bins.

- Dates
- Dried pineapple
- Dried banana chips
- Dried cherries
- Dried blueberries

Beans

Look for bulk bins or organic brands.

- Black-eyed peas
- Green lentils
- Red lentils
- Black beans
- Kidney beans
- Pinto beans
- Navy beans
- Split peas
- Popcorn

Other Protein

- Tofu
- Tempeh

Milk

- Unsweetened Silk soymilk (silksoymilk.com)
- Strawberry and banana Vitasoy soymilk (vitasoy-usa.com)
- Carob Edensoy soymilk (edenfoods.com)

Extras for Cooking

- Annie's organic yellow mustard (annies.com)
- Annie's organic horseradish mustard
- Apple cider vinegar
- Bionaturae organic extra virgin olive oil (bionaturae .com)
- Bionaturae tomato paste
- Bionaturae crushed tomatoes
- Bionaturae strained tomatoes
- Cascadian Farm pickles (cascadianfarm.com)
- Creamy and whipped Earth Balance butter (earth balance.net)
- Eden organic sauerkraut
- Herbs: fresh or dried organic basil, clove, fennel, garlic, parsley, turmeric
- Imus Ranch salsa (imusranchfoods.com)
- Imus Ranch balsamic vinaigrette
- Mediterranean Organic wild capers (mediterranean organic.com)
- Muir Glen organic ketchup (muirglen.com)
- Muir Glen fire-roasted tomatoes
- Natural Value dijon mustard (naturalvalue.com)
- Organic tamari soy sauce
- Spectrum mayonnaise (spectrumorganics.com)

- Spectrum canola oil
- Spectrum safflower oil

Sustainable Animal Products

If you do eat animal foods, your best bet is to buy from local farmers at a farmers' market, natural grocery store, or local butcher. Their meat and dairy will be the freshest, and you can ask questions about how it was raised and handled. Visit eatwellguide.org (an excellent site run by IATP and Sustainable Table, a nonprofit group that raises awareness about problems in our food supply) to find markets near you. But if local, sustainable animal products are hard to find in your area, you can try these trustworthy national brands of organic and certified humane animal products. For more suggestions, visit www.certifiedhumane.org.

Organic Dairy

- Brown Cow Farm yogurt (browncowfarm.com)
- Cowgirl Creamery cheeses (cowgirlcreamery.com)
- Horizon Organic milk, yogurt, cheeses, cream cheese, butter, ice cream, sour cream, and eggs (horizonorganic .com)
- Organic Valley Farms milk, soymilk, butter, sour cream, cheese, and cottage cheese (organicvalley.coop)
- Stonyfield Farm yogurts, milk, and ice cream (stonyfield farm.com)
- Fleur de la Terre artisan cheese (grassfedtraditions .com)

Grass-Fed Organic Beef

- Applegate Farms (nitrite-free hot dogs and lunch meats (applegatefarms.com)
- Grateful Harvest (albertsorganics.com)
- Niman Ranch (nimanranch.com)
- North Hollow Farm (vermontgrassfedbeef.com)

Certified Humane Organic Pork

- Applegate Farms bacon, cured meats, and ham
- Caw Caw Creek Farm heirloom pork, sausage, bratwurst, proscuitto, and bacon (cawcawcreek.com)
- Flying Pigs Farm (flyingpigsfarm.com)
- Niman Ranch

Certified Humane Organic Poultry

- Applegate Farms
- Alison's Family Farms chicken, turkey, and turkey bacon (alisonsfamilyfarms.com)
- Murray's Chicken (murrayschicken.com)

Fish

- EcoFish (ecofish.com)

A Greener You

Here's how eating green has helped readers like you:

About a year ago I switched to organic dairy (I drink 1-percent milk and eat low-fat vanilla yogurt) because I eat these foods every day and I have hypothyroidism, a condition where my body doesn't produce enough thyroid hormone, which can lead to a slowed metabolism and low energy. So I figured it was a good idea to take as many excess, synthetic hormones out of the picture as possible, to eliminate that confounding factor, since it's unclear what triggers hypothyroidism, and since I had to add a synthetic hormone to my body in the form of medication for my condition.

—Melissa, 30, New York, New York

I try to only buy milk and yogurt that's organic or at least hormone free. My husband and I often buy our milk at the neighborhood farmers' market from Ronnybrook Farm, a local dairy in the Hudson Valley. They're not certified organic but still rank high on the sustainability scale because they're hormone free and give their cows access to pasture for part of the year. I also like them because the milk comes in an old-fashioned bottle, which you return to them, so they can wash and reuse the bottles.

—Jen, 31, Brooklyn, New York

I stopped eating meat sixteen years ago but continued to eat dairy and eggs in limited amounts until eight months ago. Giving them up was the best decision I've ever made. I have less congestion and fewer colds. Avoiding dairy has also eliminated menstrual symptoms and improved my skin. (I used to have acne, which has now disappeared.)

—Priya, 39, Dublin, Ohio

Chapter 3

The Power of Produce

When I was growing up I ate the typical American diet—heavy on the roast beef, butter-soaked mashed potatoes, and tall glasses of milk, with maybe a few peas or carrots on the side. This is what "healthy eating" meant back then, but I never felt good. All those animal foods felt like they took forever for my body to digest. I was always congested and hoarse, suffering from allergies or colds. And as a competitive runner, I never felt that I performed as well as I wanted on a meat-based diet.

I began experimenting with a vegetarian diet in high school and college, but it wasn't until I moved to New York after college that my health really improved. It was really luck—my apartment just happened to be across the street from a health food store and restaurant. I wandered in one day because the sign said "vegetarian" and signed up for a cooking class where I learned what healthy eating is all about.

We all know there are many excellent reasons to eat more plant foods. "Eating plenty of fruits and vegetables can help you ward off heart disease and stroke, control blood pressure and cholesterol, prevent some types of cancer, avoid a painful intestinal ailment called diverticulitis, and guard against cataract and macular degeneration, two common causes of vision loss," reports the Nutrition Source, an excellent health information Web site run by Department of Nutrition researchers at the Harvard School of Public Health (www.hsph.harvard .edu/nutritionsource).

In fact, the Harvard-based Nurses' Health Study and Health Professionals Follow-Up Study, which collected data on the eating habits of almost 110,000 men and women, found that those of us who eat at least eight servings of fruits and vegetables daily are 30 percent less likely to have a heart attack or stroke than folks who average fewer than two servings per day. And the study authors concluded that for every extra serving you eat, your risk of heart disease drops another four percent. Green leafy vegetables such as lettuce, spinach, Swiss chard, and mustard greens; cruciferous vegetables such as broccoli, cauliflower, cabbage, Brussels sprouts, bok choy, and kale; and citrus fruits such as oranges, lemons, limes, and grapefruit (and their juices) seem to be the most beneficial.

In another study, called the Dietary Approaches to Stop Hypertension (DASH) trial, volunteers ate a diet rich in produce and low-fat dairy, while restricting their intake of saturated and total fat. Just by following this diet, those participants with high blood pressure were able to lower their readings as effectively as with hypertension medication. Of course in studies like these, it's impossible to know whether the benefit came from something in the vegetables themselves or because of the reduction in animal foods. Further research will sort that out, but no need for you to worry, because the benefit is clear: Eating a wide variety of fruits and vegetables ensures you're exposed to all the health-promoting compounds they contain.

Scientists have isolated a few components in fruits and vegetables that have a clear and positive effect on your health. One is their indigestible fiber. This fiber passes through your digestive system, sopping up water like a sponge, explains Nutrition Source. "This can calm the irritable bowel and by triggering regular bowel movements, can relieve or prevent constipation. The bulking and softening action of insoluble fiber also decrease pressure inside the intestinal tract and so may help prevent diverticulosis (the development of tiny, easily irritated pouches inside the colon) and diverticulitis (the often painful inflammation of these pouches)." All plant foods have fiber; apples, beans, blueberries, carrots, celery, cucumbers, dried peas, lentils, pears, strawberries, tomatoes, and zucchini are among the best sources. (Whole grains are also an excellent source—more on them in chapter 4.)

Dark green leafy vegetables also contain two pigments, lutein and zeaxanthin, which researchers now know are essential for good eye health. They appear to be able to snuff out free-radical damage (generated by sunlight, cigarette smoke, air pollution, infection, and metabolism) before it harms the eye's sensitive tissues, reports Nutrition Source. And this just scratches the surface of what we know (so far!) about the many health-protective benefits of plant foods.

So Why Aren't We Eating Enough Plants?

We know we should include more plant foods in our diets, but we just plain aren't doing it. "One-third of all vegetables consumed in the United States come from just three sources: French fries, potato chips, and iceberg lettuce," writes Marion Nestle, PhD, in her book *What to Eat: An Aisle-by-Aisle Guide to Savvy Food Choices and Good Eating.* If you don't count potatoes, Nutrition Source reports that the average American consumes just three servings of fruits and vegetables a day, when in fact most of us need three times that—nine servings, or four and a half cups of produce daily.

Obviously, our grab-and-go culture of fast food doesn't make healthy eating easy, to say nothing of our American obsession with meat. I'll admit, being vegan can be a real pain sometimes, especially when I'm eating in restaurants or traveling. I often have to hunt pretty hard to find something on a menu that doesn't have any animal products or pack my own snacks—and when it comes to eating in airports, forget it! There are so few of us making the effort to adopt a healthier diet that we haven't really created a market for these foods yet. It's coming, slowly but surely—but there's no question that, especially in the beginning, eating green will require a little extra effort on your part. "This is an issue that people have to spend a little time on," says Diane Hatz, the founder of the non-profit Sustainable Table, which co-founded the Eat Well Guide, an excellent online resource with the Institute of Agriculture and Trade Policy to help you find healthy, sustainable food.

Vegetarian cooking guru Deborah Madison agrees. "Vegetarian cooking doesn't have to be complicated, but I do think people have to commit to learning some basic skills," she says. We need to make what we eat a top priority in our lives and stop relying on grab-and-go foods, even though their convenience is addictive. "We're hooked on having someone else do the work for us and we pay in terms of taste, nutritional quality and cost," says Dr. Michael Jacobson.

But a plant-based diet may not be as pricey as you think. Economists at the United States Department of Agriculture Economic Research Service found that you can eat three fruits and four vegetables daily for as little as sixty-four cents (in 1999 dollars). "This cost is so little that even people on very low incomes could afford it," notes Dr. Nestle. Of course this depends on where you live and shop. Eating organic produce, which I'll discuss later in this chapter, often does cost more—but it's certainly not as expensive as treating our country's obesity, heart disease, and cancer epidemics. When you choose to spend your food dollars on healthy, delicious plant foods instead of hamburgers and hot dogs, you're choosing to protect your health and, as I discussed in the last chapter, the health of our planet. And by moving health up your list of priorities, you'll also increase the quality and flavor of your life.

Eat Your Veggies 101

Whether you're going vegan, vegetarian, or just cutting down on meat, you probably have some questions about how to get your new eco-health lifestyle off the ground. Below I've answered the questions I hear most often. You can find more tips online—I especially like compassionatecooks.com, 101cookbooks.com, and vegsource.com.

Q: Will I get enough protein without eating meat?

Absolutely. All plant-based foods contain protein. In fact, you're probably getting more protein than you need on a meat-based diet. The Harvard School of Public Health (HSPH) reports that you (like all adults) need about 1 gram of protein per kilogram of body weight per day to keep your body from slowly breaking down your own tissues. That works out to about 9 grams of protein per 20 pounds, or 50 to 75 grams for most average-weight adults, but the average American consumes 90 to 95 grams of protein daily, according to T. Colin Campbell, PhD, author of *The China Study*.

Although we think of protein as healthy, Dr. Campbell's research suggests that this level of excessive consumption could be dangerous and potentially linked to "heart disease, various cancers, kidney stones, gout and bone problems." The Harvard-based Nurses' Health Study found that women who ate more than 95 grams of protein per day were 20 percent more likely to have a broken wrist over a twelve-month period compared to those eating less than 68 grams daily. Atkins dieters, beware: HSPH researchers also warn that "getting too much protein can leach calcium from your bones. As your body digests protein, it releases acid into the bloodstream, which the body neutralizes by drawing calcium from the bones. Animal protein seems to cause more of this calcium leaching than vegetable protein does . . . Long-term high-protein diets should be used with caution, if at all."

Q: What are the best sources of non-animal protein?

My favorite plant protein sources are fermented soy—tempeh, which you can buy in blocks, marinate, and grill like steaks; low-sodium soy sauce, which is great over vegetables; and miso paste, which is delicious in soup or as a marinade. I also love edamame, which my son and I can eat by the bowlful! These soy foods deliver plenty of polyunsaturated fat (the good kind), fiber, vitamins, and minerals and are lower in saturated fat than animal protein, as well as naturally cholesterol free. Studies show that eating approximately 50 grams of soy protein a day in place of animal protein is associated with reducing total cholesterol levels by 3 percent—if sustained over time, that could mean up to a 20-percent reduction in your risk for cardiovascular disease.

You can also get excellent quality protein from beans, nuts, and seeds. See chapter 2 for a list of my vegan pantry staples and some delicious and easy recipes. And I'm a huge fan of quinoa and other protein-rich whole grains; more on these in chapter 4.

Q: Will I get enough calcium without dairy?

Yes. Eating a variety of collard greens, spinach, kale, broccoli, figs, almonds, oatmeal, black beans, tofu, and fortified soymilk will ensure you have plenty of calcium. You do need this essential mineral in your diet—in small amounts in the bloodstream, it plays a critical role in blood clotting, muscle contraction, heartbeat maintenance, and proper nerve function. It also makes your bones and teeth strong (99 percent of the calcium in your body is stored there, then released into the bloodstream as needed).

But, like misconceptions about protein, our conviction that the more calcium, the better, may not be true. Walter Willett, MD, chair of the Department of Nutrition at the Harvard School of Public Health, says that "500 to 700 milligrams of calcium is probably adequate." That's about what you'll get in two bowls of oatmeal, a cup of spinach plus half a cup of tofu, or two glasses of fortified soymilk.

Getting enough vitamin K is also important to getting enough calcium because it helps your body absorb the mineral properly. One or more servings per day of broccoli, Brussels sprouts, dark green lettuce, collard greens, or kale should be enough to meet the daily recommendation of 120 micrograms for men and 90 micrograms for women, says the HSPH.

Q: Are there any other vitamins I need to monitor on a plant-based diet?

For the most part, eating a plant-based diet will ensure you receive much more of the essential vitamins and minerals than if you were mostly eating meat and dairy, because fruits and vegetables are so nutrient rich. However, fortified milk is most Americans' main source of vitamin D; you should include fortified soymilk, fortified orange juice, or some fortified cereals in your diet to replace that, or—even easier— spend fifteen minutes in the sun every few days, says Dr. Campbell. "This provides all the vitamin D our bodies need."

The one nutrient you should consider taking as a supplement if you decide to give up all animal products is vitamin B_{12}. "This essential nutrient can be found in plants if they are grown in a healthy organic soil rich with microorganisms," says Dr. Campbell. But when you aren't able to eat exclusively organic produce, "supplements are necessary if no animal products are consumed. This is not a flaw in plant-based foods—it is merely a symptom of our separation from nature."

Green Your Plate

Eating green can be as simple as buying a bag of organic apples instead of a bag of chips. "All vegetables can be cooked in a simple, straightforward manner," says Deborah Madison, who gives tons of easy and tasty suggestions in her classic plant foods bible *Vegetarian Cooking for Everyone*. But to reap the maximum benefits of a plant-based diet, you need to know how your produce is grown, where it comes from—and how to choose the healthiest kind for you and your family.

Go Organic

I can't emphasize enough the importance of choosing organically grown fruits and vegetables whenever you can. According to the USDA, any fruit or vegetable carrying the USDA Organic seal has been "produced by farmers who emphasize the use of renewable resources and the conservation of soil and water to enhance environmental quality for future generations." It is also grown "without using most conventional pesticides, fertilizers made with synthetic ingredients, or sewage sludge, bioengineering, or ionizing radiation. Before a product can be labeled 'organic,' a Government-approved certifier inspects the farm where the food is grown to make sure the farmer is following all the rules necessary to meet USDA organic standards."

In one fell swoop, buying organic protects you and your family from a host of health threats. Conventional farmers spray their crops with tremendous amounts of incredibly toxic pesticides. "My feeling is these pesticides are used to kill insects, so how could they possibly be good for us?" says Dr. Marion Nestle. As she explains in *What to Eat,* "Critics say, 'So what? Pesticides are safe.' As evidence, they say that nobody has ever died from eating the small amounts of pesticide residues on food. Oh, please. Pesticides are demonstrably harmful to farm-workers and to 'nontarget' wildlife, and they accumulate in soils for ages . . . If they really were all that benign, there would be no reason for the government to bother to regulate them, but it does. Scientists may not be able to quantify the degree of harm they cause, but that does not mean that pesticides are safe for you."

Studies are beginning to emerge that document the potential risks of these toxins. Some pesticides have been associated with an increased risk for Parkinson's disease, according to a Harvard study of 140,000 people published in the August 2006 issue of *Annals of Neurology.* Researchers surveyed the group on their exposure to various chemicals in 1982 and then followed them for two decades to track who developed the disease. Those who reported pesticide exposure at work or home had a 70-percent greater incidence of Parkinson's disease than those who weren't exposed, even after controlling for exposure to environmental contaminants like asbestos and gasoline exhaust.

Who is most vulnerable to the developmental and carcinogenic risks of pesticide exposure? Our kids. One million American children age five and younger consume unsafe levels of pesticides every day, mostly from produce, according to a report by the Environmental Working Group. Apples, grapes, peaches, and pears are the most common sources of exposure to unsafe levels of these organophosphate pesticides, which can harm the developing brain and nervous system. About one apple in eight will expose a child to an unsafe dose.

Choosing organic produce is an easy way to avoid this exposure. A University of Washington study found that children eating a diet of at least 75 percent organic fruits and vegetables had concentrations of pesticide metabolites six to nine times lower than children eating 75 percent conventional produce. The difference was enough for researchers to conclude that organic fruits and vegetables can potentially reduce exposure levels from above to below the EPA's limit for chronic exposure, "thereby shifting exposures from a range of uncertain risk to a range of negligible risk."

Non-organic produce can also be contaminated with sewage sludge, which is used as fertilizer. It can contain bacteria, viruses, heavy metals, synthetic organic chemicals, prescription drug residues, lead, and pathogens such as *E. coli* and salmonella, report researchers at the Institute for Agriculture and Trade Policy.

In addition to allowing you to avoid a host of toxins, organic fruits and vegetables also offer you a huge array of health benefits. Organically grown produce tends to have higher antioxidant levels than conventionally grown produce, say University of California, Davis scientists who published their research in the *Journal of Agricultural and Food Chemistry* in 2003. Among their findings: Organic corn contained 59 percent higher levels of antioxidants, organic blackberries contained 50 percent higher, and organic strawberries contained 19 percent higher levels than their conventionally grown counterparts. A 2001 evidence review of forty-one research trials published in the *Journal of Alternative and Complementary Medicine* concluded that organic produce generally boasts 27 percent more vitamin C, 21 percent more iron, 29 percent more magnesium, and 13 percent more phosphorous than conventionally grown produce. For a list of my favorite fruits and vegetables, as well as a shopper's guide to which produce is most important to buy organic (because it harbors the most pesticide residue) see my Eating Green Guide, which starts on page 52.

Say No to Genetically Modified Organisms (GMOs)

If you buy organic produce, you'll never need to worry that it has been grown from seeds containing GMOs. But conventional produce growers are turning more and more to GM seeds that have been engineered to withstand pests and harsh growing conditions and to produce vegetables that are identical in size, shape, and taste. And growing these Frankenfruits is playing Russian roulette with our health, because for the most part we have absolutely no idea whether such genetic engineering is safe for human consumption or not. "Many industries support the development and use of GMOs while many consumers and organizations question their safety and have called for adequate and independent testing of GMO products," explains Diane Hatz of Sustainable Table. "It's legal for farmers in the U.S. and some other countries like Spain, Germany and Argentina to produce and sell certain GMOs for human and animal consumption, but some European countries are working to ban GMOs until further testing can be done to prove they are safe."

Consumer outcry has deterred many produce growers from adopting GMO plants so far. But "about 80 percent of the papayas grown in Hawaii are genetically modified to resist the ringspot virus, which nearly destroyed the Hawaiian industry for this fruit a few years ago," reports Dr. Marion Nestle. "If you buy a papaya from Hawaii, there is a good chance it is genetically modified." Look for "No GMOs" or "GMO Free" on produce stickers to ensure you're avoiding them. It's harder to know if you're getting GMOs in processed foods, but assume that you are unless the label says otherwise: In 2004, 85 percent of American soybean acres and 45 percent of corn acres were planted with genetically engineered varieties. These two crops are the basis for most hydrogenated oils and sweeteners used in processed foods today.

Look for Local

Whether it's grown organically or not, the food you buy in the grocery store has traveled an average of fifteen hundred miles to reach your table—that's about twenty-seven times farther than food you can buy at your local farmers' market, reports Hatz. About 40 percent of our fruit is grown overseas, and even though broccoli and apples are grown within twenty to sixty miles of the average American's house, they travel around seventeen hundred to eighteen hundred miles before you pick them up at your supermarket, because chain stores rely on central distribution systems to receive their stock. Well-traveled produce isn't as good for you. Fruits and vegetables are most nutritious when they're fresh because that's when vitamin, mineral, and antioxidant contents are at their peak. Produce that has taken a week to ten days to reach your refrigerator has significantly less amounts of nutrients that the produce being sold at your nearest farmers' market.

Stone Barns Center for Food and Agriculture, Polyface Farm, the Imus Ranch, and many other small, sustainable farms are "beyond organic," meaning they follow the USDA organic standards and then some. But some small farmers do use pesticides and other toxic chemicals on their crops, so when you shop at a farmers' market, it's important to ask a farmer if he uses pesticides or fertilizers before you buy (unless you see the "Certified Organic" sign displayed). Some local food advocates argue that buying from a small farmer is always better, even if he or she isn't organic. They claim that the "Big Organic" growers like Earthbound Farm, Cascadian Farm, and other brands sold at supermarket chains like Whole Foods and Wal-Mart are little better than large-scale industrial conventional farms. Their concerns are that large-scale farming of any kind is tough on the land, wastes fossil fuels, edges out smaller farmers, and ultimately may weaken our standards for what counts as organic.

I disagree. When I buy an Earthbound Farm mesclun salad mix at a New York City grocery store, the number of miles it has traveled from California troubles me. But on the other hand, Earthbound Farm has turned 40,000 acres of farmland across California, Washington, Oregon, Arizona, Colorado, Mexico, Canada, Chile, and New Zealand into pesticide-free zones. And the fact that Wal-Mart is pricing their organic foods just 10 percent higher than conventional goods means that more low-income families can afford it. Healthy eating should not be a luxury of the wealthy.

Eating Green Guide

Here's a collection of tips and resources to help you make the most of your plant-based diet. Bon appétit!

Smart Shopper Produce Guide

Some fruits and vegetables are more heavily sprayed or more likely to absorb pesticide residues than others. Researchers at the IATP culled this list (based on studies by the USDA and the Environmental Working Group) to help you minimize your pesticide exposure even if you can't buy all your produce organic. If you do have to buy conventional, thoroughly wash your produce under cold water, then scrub potatoes, peel carrots, stem strawberries, and so on. Washing reduced the amount of pesticide residue on produce in half in one study and where residues remained, levels declined significantly after washing, reports the IATP.

Highest Pesticide Residue

- Apples
- Bell and hot peppers
- Carrots
- Celery
- Cherries

- Grapes (imported)
- Green beans
- Nectarines
- Peaches
- Pears
- Potatoes
- Red raspberries
- Spinach
- Strawberries

Moderate Pesticide Residue

- Apricots
- Blueberries
- Cantaloupe
- Collard greens
- Cucumbers
- Grapes (domestic)
- Honeydew melons
- Kale
- Lettuce
- Mushrooms
- Oranges
- Sweet potatoes

- Tomatoes
- Turnip greens
- Winter squash

Least Pesticide Residue

- Apple juice
- Asparagus
- Avocados
- Bananas
- Broccoli
- Cabbage
- Cauliflower
- Kiwi
- Mangoes
- Onions
- Orange juice
- Papayas
- Pineapple
- Plums
- Sweet corn
- Sweet peas
- Tangerines
- Watermelon

How to Find Your Farmers' Market

These Web sites will guide you to farmers' markets, farm stands, and stores stocking local, sustainably grown food in your area:

- www.localharvest.org
- www.eatwellguide.org
- www.ams.usda.gov/farmersmarkets

Label Lingo

"Certified Organic" is by the far the most important labels to look for on your fruits and vegetables. But these other labels are also good indicators that the food you're about to buy was grown in the most environmentally friendly circumstances possible.

- **Northeast Eco-Apple Project.** Apple orchards from northeastern states can use this seal if they have met standards set by the IPM Institute, a nonprofit integrated pest management organization. The criteria include ensuring worker safety and using less toxic pesticides. For more info, visit www.ipminstitute.org

- **Fair Trade Certified.** This label is monitored and awarded by TransFair USA to ensure farmers receive fair prices and that environmentally friendly, worker-safe practices were used. You'll see it on bananas and other tropical fruit as well as coffee, tea, chocolate, rice, and sugar. Visit www.transfairusa.org.

- **Wisconsin Healthy Grown Potatoes.** This label, which has been recognized by the USDA and the World

Wildlife Fund, appears on potatoes from Wisconsin farmers who have been vetted to ensure they are using fewer, less toxic pesticides and more sustainable farming practices. Visit www.healthygrown.com.

Eco Shopping List

Here's a list of my favorite fruits and vegetables, plus ideas on what to do with them.

- **Avocados.** It's a misconception that these are too fattening—they're rich in the healthy monounsaturated and polyunsaturated fats that we need in our diet, as well as vitamin E. I like to cut them in half and eat them with a spoon for breakfast—they're so rich and creamy, they don't need any preparation! But they are also delicious sliced in a sandwich with some lettuce, tomato, salt, and balsamic vinegar. And see my guacamole recipe on page 238.

- **Berries.** Fresh or dried, I can't get enough of cherries, strawberries, blueberries, and goji berries (a Tibetan fruit available in health food stores) because they're high in antioxidants and absolutely delicious. I like to mix a handful of dried cherries or goji berries with a handful of green pistachio nuts—I call it my Christmas snack!

- **Japanese sweet potatoes.** These are smaller, longer, and skinnier than regular sweet potatoes, are packed with nutrients, and have a dark purple skin and deep orange flesh. You can find them at Asian supermarkets or gourmet food stores. Scrub them clean, then brush the skin lightly with olive oil, sprinkle with sea salt and bake for thirty to forty minutes on 400 degrees Fahrenheit. They're so yummy and creamy, my husband and I love to eat them hot or cold as snacks.

- **Jicama.** I call this white vegetable the Southwestern Cucumber because it has the same cooling properties as regular cucumbers, which are so good for digestion. I like to cut them up and eat them like carrot sticks or toss slices of jicama with lemon juice, olive oil, and parsley for a delicious salad.

- **Kale.** There are several different varieties of kale and they're all delicious and easy to prepare. Just wash it thoroughly, chop it up, and throw it in a wok or stainless steel pan with some safflower oil, sea salt, and minced garlic. Sauté it for no more than a minute or two—you want it to stay crisp and vibrant green—then serve it as a nutritious side dish to any meal.

A Greener You

Check out why these readers are switching to a plant-based diet:

Being vegan has also opened up a whole new spectrum of tastes for me. I am excited to try new products and new recipes. I eat non–genetically modified soy products, such as soymilk, tofu, and tempeh. I also eat a lot of beans and lentils, as well as nuts. I try to consume a variety of vegetables and also use a variety of grains such as rice, spelt, and quinoa. I am lactose intolerant and my health has improved tremendously since switching to all plant foods.

—Priya, 39, Dublin, Ohio

My mother and I often commiserate lately over the lack of people who cook with real ingredients. More and more often I'll be at the grocery store unloading my cart with bread, pastas, vegetables, and fresh herbs, and the people in front or behind me will be eating all packaged, frozen, microwave foods.

I'm a journalist just one year out of college, so I certainly understand that it's cheap to eat that way. But I think it's actually more efficient to cook with vegetables (I buy from my farmers' market and choose organic whenever fiscally possible) than not cook at all. I started learning to cook my last year at school and found it to be relaxing and healthy. It also wasn't as difficult as I anticipated—as my mother always says, "If you can read, you can cook." I now live with my boyfriend and we both appreciate the cost, taste, and healthfulness of eating real food from a grill or stovetop and not from a cardboard box or microwave.

—Cara, 23, Fort Collins, Colorado

I became vegetarian seven years ago, and am now in fact moving toward a more vegan diet. The health benefits are enormous and obvious. My husband and I, as well as our eight-year-old grandson who lives with us, haven't been sick in a very long time and take no medications. It's not only helped my cholesterol and my weight—it's also helped my food budget. I save money because I'm not buying meats anymore.

We get plenty of protein by eating beans, grains like quinoa, soy products, nuts, or eggs. As for fruits and vegetables, we grow almost all of our own and after five years have built our soil and our gardening skills to the point that we're able to produce enough during our growing season here in the mountains of northeastern Tennessee to keep us supplied all year, by preserving them through canning, freezing, or drying. I sincerely believe that building up my soil using organic compost, rock powders, manures, and green cover crops provides us with many more nutrients than one would ordinarily find in grocery-store produce.

—Jan, 54, Johnson City, Tennessee

Chapter 4

Out of the Box:
Snacks and Processed Foods

By the time I got to college I was a pretty committed vegetarian and on my way to phasing out all animal products, in order to be a true vegan. But as a college student and even into my early twenties, I wouldn't say I was a healthy vegan, because I didn't really understand how to make a plant-based diet work for me. In fact, I think I was very unhealthy for many years because I hadn't learned how to eat correctly. I chose salads, but they weren't much more than iceberg lettuce, cucumbers, and maybe a tomato, all coated in bottled salad dressing full of fat and sugar. I also ate a lot of processed snacks—I thought if I bought banana chips or a carob bar at the health food store, it must be good for me! This was in the late 1980s, when good organic fruits and vegetables weren't widely available and health food stores mostly just stocked packaged foods or those mysterious bulk binned items.

But it wasn't just that healthy foods were hard to find back then. Almost everyone who switches to a plant-based diet today still struggles to figure out what "healthy eating" really means. "Just being a vegetarian or a vegan doesn't guarantee that you're going to have a great diet," says the Center for Science in the Public Interest's Dr. Michael Jacobson.

"Lots of vegetarians, especially teenagers, live on Hostess Twinkies and soda pop. Technically those foods are vegan, because they don't contain animal products—but they certainly aren't good for you."

Our grab-and-go culture, where breakfast is a doughnut you gulp down as you're fighting traffic, lunch is at a fast food restaurant, and dinner is a bowl of cereal eaten standing over the sink, just doesn't make eating well easy. In fact, many of us are so busy that the idea of three square meals a day has gone out the window, and we race around subsisting mostly on snacks. In *What to Eat,* Dr. Marion Nestle notes that more than 80 percent of Americans snack at least once a day. Sodas and juice drinks are the most popular choice, but the proportion of our daily calories that comes from salty snacks has doubled.

It's no wonder: The food industry introduces about twenty thousand new products into supermarkets each year, she reports—approximately three thousand candies, three thousand snack foods, two thousand sodas and juice drinks, one thousand baked goods, and more than one hundred new versions of breakfast cereals. These companies' marketers claim they're trying to help you fit nutritious meals into your busy lifestyle. But the middle aisles of every grocery store in the country are bursting with candies, chips, cookies, sodas, and other junk, all of which are loaded with way too much sugar, fat, and salt, not to mention synthetic chemical additives that are harmful to your health.

I'm including this chapter on processed foods because I know that simply reducing your meat consumption isn't enough to improve your health, let alone lighten your eco footprint (about 1.8 million tons of food packaging clogs our landfills each year; we also dispose of 3.3 million tons of plastic bags and 3.5 billion pounds of lunchbox garbage). If you really want to eat green you also have to cut this junk out of your diet. I promise you won't starve—if you're shopping at your farmers' market and filling your fridge with delicious organic fruits and vegetables, it will be a snap to replace unhealthy, processed meals with whole foods that taste great because they're packed with nutrients. But you'll have an easier time just saying no to junk food if you know a little bit about how marketers trick us into eating so much of it and exactly what it is these foods contain that make them taste so good—but wreak havoc on your health.

The "Healthy Junk Food" Trap

As Michael Pollan says, we're an unhealthy nation obsessed with learning how to eat better. And as we struggle to fit nutrition into our time-crunched lives, the idea of healthy fast food seems like the Holy Grail. "[Food manufacturers] know that you are more likely to buy processed foods if you think they are good for you," says Dr. Marion Nestle. "So they go way beyond enrichment and put all kinds of additional vitamins and minerals into everything they can—and then boast of the nutritional value of those additives on the packaging." If you believe everything you read, then practically every snack in those center grocery store aisles is "part of a nutritious breakfast," lunch, and dinner. Some processed foods are worse than others, of course, depending on the amount of calories and the ingredients they contain. But anytime you eat something out of a box or a wrapper, no matter what health claims the manufacturer is making, view it as a treat. If you're eating it for breakfast, lunch, or dinner, know that you could be getting many more nutrients for the calories if you were eating a whole food instead.

Food Additives to Avoid

Of course I know it's impossible for you to live your life without ever eating another processed food. Chances are good that sometimes you'll find yourself trapped in an airport, on a long car trip, or just in need of a once in a blue moon treat after a long day at work. In fact, I think the occasional indulgence is important. If you tell yourself you'll never eat doughnuts again, you probably won't last a week without giving in—and eating a whole box. The truth is, if you're consistently eating a healthy diet most of the time, then enjoying the occasional junk doughnut or slice of pizza won't kill you. But—especially if you find yourself eating these foods more often—you should know what you're eating. Here are the most common and most harmful additives that pop up on ingredient lists in the processed food aisles.

1. Bad Fats

Of course you know by now that not all fats are evil. The healthy list includes monounsaturated, polyunsaturated, omega-3s, and omega-6s. You need these in your diet to maintain good health, but they are readily available in plant foods like avocados, seeds, and nuts, so don't buy a snack because the label touts its healthy fat content. Chances are the manufacturer just threw in a dose of omega-3s to distract you from the rest of the ingredient label. More often, processed foods contain little to none of these good fats, and plenty of the following unhealthy kinds:

Saturated Fat

Because this fat is so prevalent in meat and dairy foods, I've already discussed its ability to increase heart disease risk in chapter 2. Plant-based foods have much lower levels, of course, but when they're turned into processed snacks, the saturated fat content can skyrocket. (Just compare a regular potato to a bag of potato chips!) The American Heart Association says that we should limit our saturated fat intake to no more than 7 percent of our daily calories. If you eat about 2,000 calories a day, that means a max of 16 grams (or 144 calories) of saturated fat per day. To keep your consumption in check, the Center for Science in the Public Interest suggests avoiding packaged foods containing more than 1.5 grams of saturated fat per serving.

Trans Fatty Acids

Trans fats are formed when liquid oils (usually soybean) are turned into solid fats through a process known as hydrogenation. You'll find these fats in shortening, margarine, crackers, cookies, candy, fried foods, and other processed foods. "It is now well established that trans fats raise levels of low-density lipoprotein ("bad") cholesterol, increasing the risk of heart disease," reports the *Green Guide,* an online publication of the National Geographic Society. Harvard School of Public Health researchers estimate that trans fat has been causing about fifty thousand premature heart attack deaths each year.

It used to be the only way you could tell if a food contained trans fat was if it listed partially hydrogenated vegetable oil on the ingredient list. But in 2006 the Food and Drug Administration decided to require food manufacturers to list trans fat content on nutrition information panels. The U.S. Department of Agriculture recommends keeping trans fat consumption as low as possible, while the American Heart Association advises not to let trans fat exceed 1 percent of your total daily calories, or about 2 grams per day.

2. Salt

Dr. Michael Jacobson's team at the Center for Science in the Public Interest describes salt as "probably the single most dangerous ingredient in our food supply." It's added to every kind of processed food you can imagine—chips, crackers, cookies, granola bars, candy, frozen dinners, juice drinks, and so on—because it "heightens flavors, reduces bitterness, and enhances sweetness," notes Dr. Marion Nestle. "It is cheap. It keeps food from becoming discolored, and it extends shelf life."

As a result, we're eating about twice as much salt as is healthy, with 70 to 90 percent of the 3,500 to 4,000 milligrams the average American consumes daily coming from processed foods and restaurant meals. Health organizations recommend keeping your salt intake to no more than a teaspoon, or 2,000 to 2,400 milligrams per day (1,500 milligrams for seniors) because too much can cause your blood pressure to skyrocket. About 65 million Americans currently suffer from high blood pressure, while another 45 million have prehypertension (elevated blood pressure levels that can lead to cardiovascular disease if left unchecked), so the CSPI calculates that halving the salt content in processed and restaurant foods would save 150,000 lives a year in the United States. The easiest way to monitor your salt intake is to limit processed foods or at least choose those labeled "low salt" or "reduced sodium."

3. Sugars

Whether it's called sugar, sucrose, dextrose, honey, fruit concentrate, fructose, corn syrup, high fructose corn syrup, or a host of other names, and whether it's derived from sugarcane, sugar beets, fruit, or corn, every gram of sugar adds four calories but zero nutritional value to your food. These kinds of refined sugars are quickly digested, which means they cause your blood glucose levels to spike and then fall rapidly. As a result you feel hungry again quite quickly (your body signals you to eat when your blood glucose levels need replenishing), which may cause you to overeat. Do this often enough and over time the excess glucose in your system can put you at risk for diabetes and heart disease. On average, Dr. Nestle reports that we're now eating thirty-one teaspoons of sugar per day—seventeen from corn syrups and fourteen from sucrose, the common table sugar refined from sugarcane and sugar beets. This adds up to five hundred empty calories per day, or about 25 percent of your average daily caloric needs.

Of all the sugars added to snack foods, high fructose corn syrup (HFCS) receives the most media scrutiny. Part of the reason is that it has become so ubiquitous. It pops up in everything from salad dressings to mustard to breads, as well as the more obvious candy bars and cookies. There are also some nutrition experts who believe HFCS is the real culprit behind the obesity epidemic because our bodies process it differently than other kinds of sugar. "Fructose does not provide the 'satiety' signals to the brain that glucose [blood sugar] does," reports the *Green Guide*. "Some experts also theorize that HFCS causes the liver to release more fat into the bloodstream. This makes people feel they want to eat more, even as they are storing up more fat." But the evidence behind these claims is spotty at best. "The critics of HFCS have absolutely no scientific basis for their contention that it's more harmful than regular sugar," says Dr. Jacobson. "People should avoid consuming too much refined sugar, including regular and HFCS, because it adds empty calories, promotes obesity and tooth decay, and may squeeze healthier foods out of your diet."

The bottom line on sugars of any kind is that they should not exceed 10 percent of your daily 2,000 calories, or about 60 grams (4 tablespoons) per day. Of course it's easy to reach that amount from the naturally occurring sugars found in all whole foods. But there's no reason to worry about natural sugar—whole grains, fruits, and vegetables also contain plenty of fiber, which will slow your digestion and prevent your blood glucose from spiking, as well as many vitamins, minerals, and other nutrients you need. It's the *added* sugars in processed foods that you want to avoid. Unfortunately, the FDA does not require manufacturers to tell you how much of a food's sugar content is added and how much is naturally occurring. A good rule of thumb: "If a food has 15 grams of sugar or more per serving, you can consider it a dessert and treat it as such," advises Dr. Nestle.

4. Artificial Sweeteners

Want to avoid added sugars? Food-industry logic says you should turn to calorie-free artificial sweeteners instead. But unless you're diabetic and can't process regular sugar, these chemical concoctions may be worse for you than the real thing—after all, their use has risen alongside the rate of obesity. When you think you're getting something (a tasty treat, a refreshing beverage, even a whole meal) for nothing (calorie free!), more often than not you'll eat twice as much or make up the calories elsewhere in your diet. But what really concerns me about artificial sweeteners is that they may increase your risk for cancer. I prefer to avoid foods containing these altogether and sweeten my whole foods as needed with agave nectar, stevia, maple syrup (grade B), evaporated cane juice, brown rice syrup (I like Lundberg's Sweet Dreams brand, www.lundberg.com), or organic chocolate syrup (I love Ah!laska's, www.ahlaska.com).

Aspartame

The Center for Science in the Public Interest says, "The bottom line is that lifelong consumption of aspartame [sold commercially as NutraSweet] probably increases the risk of cancer. People—especially young children—should not consume foods and beverages sweetened with [it]." Though there are critics of this position, Jacobson's team based their conclusion on a 2007 study by researchers at the Ramazzini Foundation in Bologna, Italy, where rats exposed to aspartame in utero had increased rates of leukemias, lymphomas, and breast cancer over the course of three years. Some of the rats developed cancer after consuming as little as 20 milligrams of aspartame per pound of body weight—the equivalent of an 150-pound adult drinking seven and a half cans of diet soda per day. Sounds like a lot, but it's actually far less than the FDA's acceptable daily limit of 50 milligrams of aspartame per kilogram of weight per day. And even if you don't drink that much soda, you may encounter aspartame in hundreds of other products (see below). Critics of the study claim that it has certain flaws, but it is clearly cause for concern.

Found In: "Diet" foods, including soft drinks, drink mixes, gelatin desserts, puddings, low-calorie frozen desserts, some ice pops, "light" yogurts, reduced-sugar gums, candies, Kool-Aid, and Equal packets.

Saccharin

Food companies love to use this sweetener because it's 350 times sweeter than sugar. But the CSPI reports that many studies on animals have shown that saccharin can cause cancer of the urinary tract, uterus, ovaries, skin, blood vessels, and other organs. A survey by the National Cancer Institute found that the use of both saccharin and cyclamate (another artificial sweetener, now banned by the FDA) was associated with a higher incidence of bladder cancer, though it could not determine a cause-and-effect relationship. The FDA has removed saccharin from its "Report on Carcinogens," but many experts believe that the evidence of its safety is at best inconclusive.

Found In: Diet foods, soft drinks, Sweet'N Low packets.

Sucralose

Sold as Splenda, sucralose is actually made from sugar, which is chlorinated with phosgene, a poison gas, to make its sugar content difficult to metabolize so you don't absorb its calories. There's not much data on health effects at this time, but Whole Foods Markets refuses to carry Splenda products "because sucralose is not metabolized and, therefore, could be potentially unsafe, is more than minimally processed, and is ideologically incompatible with the company's philosophy of selling 'the highest quality natural and organic products available,'" writes Dr. Nestle.

Found In: Baked goods, diet soft drinks and juices, Splenda packets. Also sold in bags (like bags of sugar) as a cooking and baking substitute.

5. Potassium Bromate

Commercial bread makers add this chemical to increase volume and to produce bread with a fine crumb structure (the noncrust part of the loaf). Bromate causes cancer in animals, reports the CSPI, though most of it rapidly breaks down in the cooking process to form innocuous bromide. The CSPI petitioned the FDA to ban the additive in 1999 on the grounds that the tiny traces that remain in finished bread could pose a small risk to consumers. The FDA has yet to act, though the chemical has been banned in virtually every other country around the globe except Japan.

6. Propyl Gallate

This antioxidant is used as a preservative in vegetable oil, meat products, potato sticks, chicken soup base, and chewing gum. Propyl gallate retards the spoilage of fats and oils, but the best available studies on rats and mice suggest (but do not prove) it may cause cancer, says the CSPI. Although the risks to humans are a matter of some dispute, many consumer advocates suggest avoiding propyl gallate.

7. Artificial Colorings

Not all artificial colors are dangerous, but I avoid them whenever possible because it's the most obvious sign that you're about to eat something of very low nutritional value—natural, whole foods have plenty of their own color, no additives required! Here are the ones the CSPI recommends you avoid:

- **Blue No. 1.** It has been inadequately tested for safety, but preliminary research suggests a small cancer risk.

  Found In: Beverages, candy, baked goods.

- **Blue No. 2.** One study suggested (but did not prove) that this dye causes brain tumors in male mice.

  Found In: Pet food, beverages, and candy.

- **Green No. 3.** Even the industry-sponsored study suggested that this color causes bladder cancer; as a result it is rarely used, though the FDA concluded it was safe.

  Found In: Candy, beverages.

- **Red No. 3.** There's convincing evidence that this dye causes thyroid tumors in rats, according to a 1983 review committee report requested by the FDA, but a ban was overruled.

  Found In: Cherries in fruit cocktail, candy, baked goods.

- **Yellow No. 6.** This dye is the third most widely used, but industry-sponsored animal studies indicate that it can cause tumors of the adrenal gland and kidney, as well as occasional allergic reactions.

Found In: Beverages, sausages, baked goods, candy, and gelatin.

Green Your Snacks

Now that you know what ingredients to avoid on food labels, let's talk about the pros and cons of the foods themselves. It almost goes without saying that candy, cookies, chips, fast food, and other junk food should be considered once in a blue moon treats. At my house, we let my son Wyatt have pizza or another favorite junk food maybe once a month or once every two weeks. I personally find that the longer I live a vegan lifestyle, the less I actually want the occasional processed treat. When you do have a craving for something sugary or salty, satisfy it by having the real thing.

Your once in a blue moon might come more or less often than mine—don't stress about it too much. "There's a huge difference between eating junk every day and eating it once a week, and there's a pretty big difference between eating it once a week and just once a month," says Dr. Nestle. "But it's really only the every day stuff you need to worry about."

Whenever possible, you're better off having whole foods in place of these processed items. But all breads, cereals, and even frozen dinners are not created equal, so within each category I'll tell you what you need to know to make the healthiest choices.

1. Grains

Grains are plant-based foods, so you would be forgiven for thinking that makes them automatically healthy, especially since they form the base of the USDA food pyramid, and we generally eat quite a lot of them, especially wheat.

Unfortunately, the vast majority of these foods are made from refined wheat, also known as white flour. Any grain can be refined (though wheat is the most common); this means the grain seed has been milled to remove its outer layers of bran and germ, leaving just the starchy endosperm. Refined white flour has more calories than whole-wheat flour because it's more concentrated, but it has just 55 percent of the folic acid, 43 percent of the calcium, 25 percent of the iron, 17 percent of the niacin, and 13 percent of the vitamin B_6 found in whole-wheat flour. Most mills then "enrich" the white flour by adding back these nutrients, but whole grains still contain far more fiber, protein, magnesium, potassium, and other nutrients than their refined counterparts.

The health benefits of whole grains are well documented. Their fiber content plays a role in healthy digestion. And among the 34,000 women who participated in the Iowa Women's Health Study from 1986 to 2003, those who reported eating at least one serving of whole grains per day had a 30- to 36-percent lower risk of heart disease than those who ate no whole grains. In the Harvard-based Nurses' Health Study, those who ate around three servings of whole grains daily also had a 36-percent lower risk of stroke than those who ate none. While these study authors can't know for sure if the whole grain had the effect or if women who eat whole grains are also engaging in other heart-healthy behaviors (like exercising and not smoking), preliminary research suggests that people who consume at least three servings of whole grains a day have a 20- to 30-percent lower risk of developing diabetes than those who eat just one serving a week.

Whole grains, in fact, are so lightly processed, they don't really belong in a chapter about processed foods. They are an essential part of a healthy plant-based diet. I always keep brown rice, wild rice, whole-wheat pasta, rice pasta, and soba noodles on hand, as these are easy foundations for any meal. But here are a few of my other favorite whole grains, which you might not be so familiar with:

Barley

You'll see two types of this hearty, earthy grain for sale: whole-grain hulled barley, which has high levels of bran and 6.2 grams of fiber per serving, but requires a patient ninety minutes to cook, and pearled barley, which has been stripped of more of the plant's tough bran layer, but still has more fiber (3 grams per serving) than most truly refined grains and cooks in under an hour. Barley is wonderful to use instead of Arborio rice (which is a refined grain with just 2 grams of fiber per serving) in risottos.

Bulgur

At nearly 6 grams of fiber per cup, bulgur (wheat kernels that have been boiled, dried, and cracked) will do more to keep you regular than any other grain on the market. It's also a great source of antioxidants that fight free-radical damage. I like to whip it into a tasty tabbouleh salad for a quick dinner—it cooks in the same time as pasta (about ten minutes), or look for quick-cook bulgur, which only needs to be soaked in hot water for 30 minutes, not boiled.

Millet

It's crazy to me that this grain is used mostly just for birdseed, when it's one of the healthiest foods you could eat! One cup gives you 25 to 30 percent of your daily intake of magnesium, manganese, and phosphorous, as well as 6 grams of protein, 2 grams of fiber, and 122 micrograms of lutein, an antioxidant that promotes eye health. Depending on how you cook it, millet can be creamy like mashed potatoes or fluffy like rice. Cooked millet makes a great porridge-like hot breakfast cereal. I also like to buy ground millet flour to use in baking.

Oats

You're probably familiar with oats thanks to Quaker Oats products and of course oatmeal. But keep in mind that most quick-cooking oats have been refined and are no longer whole grains. Check the label—one cup of uncooked oats should contain about 8 grams of fiber and 13 grams of protein, along with 68 percent of your daily requirement for manganese, more than 25 percent of your daily selenium, and almost 20 percent of your daily thiamin (vitamin B_1). I keep whole-grain oat flour on hand for baking and love to make hearty oatmeal mixed with soymilk and topped with nuts, fruit, and a little agave sweetener for breakfast. In fact, my family enjoys this dish so much, we often have it for dinner too!

Quinoa

A hands-down favorite, quinoa contains about 23 grams of carbs and 2 grams of fiber per serving, is also high in copper and magnesium, and packs 4.5 grams of complete protein, as it's one of the few plant foods to contain all nine of the essential amino acids our bodies can't make on their own. Quinoa cooks quickly (10 to 15 minutes). I like to use it in place of rice in a pilaf or to stuff roasted peppers. Just be sure to rinse the dry quinoa before you cook it to remove a naturally occurring bitter residue of a substance called "saponins," which the plant uses to deter bugs.

Spelt

Two ounces of spelt flour gives you 76 percent of your daily riboflavin, 62 percent of your daily manganese, and almost 25 percent of your daily thiamin. Its high riboflavin content may help prevent headaches if you suffer from migraines; it's also a great source of niacin, which is associated with lowering cholesterol and preventing atherosclerosis (hardening of the arteries). Spelt flour works well in muffin and waffle recipes. I'm also a fan of spelt breads and spelt pastas—they taste much better than some of the whole-wheat pastas on the market.

Processed Grains

Whenever possible, choose whole-grain bread, pasta, cereal, and so on over refined, and feel free to experiment with these alternative grains in place of wheat and rice. But sometimes, that's easier said than done. Here's what you need to know.

Cereals

Almost every breakfast cereal on the market broadcasts its vitamin, mineral, and fiber content, even though most are heavily processed, containing a ton of additives and several teaspoons of sugar per serving. The vitamins and minerals are only there because the manufacturer has added them back into the cereal's refined flour base. With whole grains becoming the newest health craze, they're starting to add these back in too, or mixing whole and refined—either way, you lose out, nutrition-wise, compared to a bowl of whole-grain oatmeal or millet.

The good news: Healthier cereals are available in your supermarket, they're just tucked away on the highest shelves, while the junk food cereal companies pay for the privilege of targeting you right at eye level. To be sure you're buying a healthy brand, look for a short ingredient list (no additives or dyes) with a whole grain listed first. The sugar content should not exceed 15 grams per serving. Meanwhile, the fiber content should be at least 2 grams per serving—preferably more. Of course you should buy an organic brand whenever possible, to minimize exposure to pesticides and promote more environmentally friendly food production.

My Favorites. When I have some time, I like to make oatmeal or buckwheat pancakes for breakfast. On days when we're in a rush, I mix dried fruits (I like cherries, pineapple, and banana, but pick your favorites!) with almonds, walnuts, sunflower seeds, ground flax, and soymilk for a do-it-yourself, no-bake kind of granola. Another quick option is mochi organic sweet brown rice puffs, which make a delicious dairy-free, gluten-free breakfast. They come in large squares, so cut them into one-and-a-half-inch pieces and bake at 450 degrees Fahrenheit for eight to ten minutes until they puff up and are brown and crispy on the outside and chewy inside. Serve plain or with some organic soymilk, soy yogurt, or organic grapes (grainaissance.com). For more delicious ideas, see the Imus Ranch Recipes on pages 242–243.

Breads

Even when you go whole grain, supermarket breads tend to have frighteningly long ingredient lists that can include partially hydrogenated soybean oil (trans fat alert!), Splenda and other artificial sweeteners, high fructose corn syrup, molasses, honey, as well as a ton of preservatives, dyes, and dough conditioners to keep the bread soft and fresh. I prefer to buy my bread from the farmers' market, where you can get delicious, homemade loaves made with just organic whole-grain flour, yeast, and salt. This is a great opportunity to experiment with grains besides wheat—rye, millet, oat, and spelt all make delicious breads. If you do buy your bread from the supermarket, look for one labeled 100 percent whole grain (whole-grain flour will also be listed as the first ingredient) with a short ingredient list and at least 2 grams of fiber per ounce.

My Favorites. Some store-bought brands that I do trust and always keep on hand are Ezekiel 4:9 organic sprouted flourless 100% whole grain breads (foodforlife.com) and Rudy's organic sourdough and rosemary olive bread, which we use to make garlic bread for Italian meals. (Look for them at Whole Foods and other health food stores.) Both of these keep well in the freezer for months.

2. Beverages

On average, Americans drink a fifth of their total calories each day. Because these drinks don't fill us up, we usually forget that sodas, juices, shakes, and even coffee (especially those fancy blender coffee drinks!) and teas have calories. Usually they also have long lists of ingredients as well, most of which are sugars or artificial sweeteners, artificial colors, and other additives. I can't recommend it enough: Stay away from these! Or at the very least, treat them as a once in a blue moon treat. Drink water instead—it's calorie, sugar, and additive free. If you want flavor, try adding a slice of lemon or lime or some fresh-cut herbs (mint is delicious). If you do drink juice, look for 100 percent organic fruit juice that has retained its pulp (that's where most of the nutrients are found) and is additive free. You can cut calories and reduce tartness by mixing it with water.

My Favorites. Lakewood 100% pure organic pineapple juice (lakewoodjuices.com), Bionaturae organic nectars (strawberry, sicilian lemon, and wildberry, at bionaturae.com), R. W. Knudsen Just Black Cherry juice and R. W. Knudsen Very Veggie low sodium organic juice (knudsenjuices.com). All of these contain nothing but fruit and water. I also drink a ton of water and herbal tea—watermelon and chamomile are some of my favorites, wonderful for relieving stress.

3. Frozen Foods

Americans spent almost $7 billion on frozen meals in 2004, reports Dr. Nestle; $1.2 billion on frozen Italian dinners, $508 million for frozen Mexican, and nearly $300 million for frozen pot pies. We also buy plenty of frozen snacks, spending another $7 billion on ice cream and ice pops, $64 million on frozen bagels, and $3 million on frozen cookie dough. Most of these products contain sky-high levels of salt, fat, and sugar, as well as tons of "cosmetics—dyes to make the product look like real food (FD&C colors, beta-carotene and annatto); milk additives, soy oils, and thickeners . . . and emulsifiers and stabilizers to hold the whole thing together," writes Dr. Nestle. In other words, you're better off cooking ahead and freezing your own meals to reheat when you need dinner on the table fast. If you do buy frozen foods, look for organic brands with the shortest possible ingredient lists.

But come winter, the freezer aisle at your grocery store is well worth visiting for frozen fruit and vegetables. Frozen produce is picked at peak ripeness and flash frozen, so it's often much higher quality (and more nutritious) than the so-called fresh fruits and vegetables that are more than a week old, having been trucked thousands of miles to your supermarket. Just make sure you're buying organic whenever possible and check that the ingredient list doesn't include any added salt, sugar, or other preservatives.

My Favorites: I keep my freezer stocked with frozen berries and vegetables (Cascadian Farm is a great organic brand; cascadianfarm. com). Occasionally we'll have an Amy's organic pizza—I like their rice crust spinach and roasted vegetable pizzas, which have nondairy soy cheese (amys.com).

Eco Shopping List

Whole-Food Snacks

These healthy, delicious whole foods will satisfy your snack attacks without the junk.

- **Organic Apples.** "I buy a bag of the littlest apples I can find, then leave them out on the kitchen counter and grab one whenever I'm hungry," says cookbook author Deborah Madison. Apples have crunch and a tangy flavor that's a good substitute for salty chips or pretzels. If you don't like apples, try bananas, apricots, kiwis, or any other fresh or dried fruits you enjoy.

- **Organic Yogurt.** I prefer soy, but reduced-fat organic dairy yogurt is also a good option. Choose plain to avoid the added sugars and other chemicals that are dumped into most flavored kinds, then sweeten with a little agave nectar or sliced fruit. Stir in a spoonful of ground flax for added nutrients. "What's better than that?" says chef Dan Barber.

- **Edamame.** Wyatt and I can eat these soybeans by the bowlful, and they're so good for you!

- **Olives and Tofu.** Mix chunks of tofu (soy cheese works too) with a handful of black, red, or green olives. Also great with Edward and Sons' Brown Rice Snaps (edward andsons.com).

- **Almond Butter.** Spread on a slice of Ezekiel 4:9 bread, this is just delicious. Organic peanut butter, macadamia nut butter, and cashew butter are also fun to try. Top with sliced bananas, strawberries, or peaches for a quick fruit serving.

- **DIY Granola.** I mix organic dry rolled oats with walnuts, almonds, raisins, dried pineapples, blueberries, or cherries. You can experiment with the nuts, grains, and fruits you like to customize your own! Or see page 243 for my Rio Grande Granola.

- **Tofu "Cheese" Salad.** Cut up organic tofu mozzarella-style, in chunks, and combine with fresh tomatoes and Greek olives.

- **Pita Breadsticks.** Cut spelt-bread pita into strips, brush them with olive oil, then sprinkle salt, pepper, and soy parmesan cheese on top. Bake at 350 degrees Fahrenheit for ten minutes or until crispy and crunchy.

- **Yellow Rice.** Cook jasmine rice with lots of turmeric powder for a natural antioxidant meal.

Store-Bought Snacks

Quite a few companies make some very healthful, nourishing snacks that I like to have on hand for those times when we're running low on fresh foods.

- **Edward and Sons Brown Rice Snaps.** These come in yummy flavors like vegetable, cheddar, toasted onion, salsa, and black sesame, and are all organic (edwardand sons.com)

- **Late July Classic Rich or Classic Saltine Crackers.** Excellent with organic almond butter and an organic kosher dill pickle (latejuly.com).

- **Mary's Gone Crackers.** I love the caraway seeds (marysgonecrackers.com).

- **New Morning Honey Graham Crackers.** These delicious snacks are made with organic grains and no hydrogenated oils. Two full graham crackers and some organic tamari almonds make a delicious snack (mannaharvest.net).

- **NuGo Organic Bars.** A fun treat, because these come in lots of great flavors like orange smoothie and banana chocolate (nugonutrition.com).

- **Oskri Organics Sesame Seed Bars.** These contain brown rice, are very high in iron, and come in a variety of flavors: molasses, date syrup and black cumin, date syrup and fennel, molasses and fennel, and molasses and black cumin (oskri.com).

Once in a Blue Moon Favorites

Everyone needs to indulge every now and then. Here are some of my favorite treats:

- **Root Beer Floats.** I love Virgil's root beer, which is sweetened only with iron-rich molasses and is a great alternative to junky sodas. It's a refreshing blend of anise, licorice, vanilla, cinnamon, clove, wintergreen, sweet birch, molasses, nutmeg, pimento berry oil, balsam oil, and oil of cassia, and it's gluten free too. To make floats, put two scoops of vanilla Soy Delicious ice cream in a parfait glass or tall drinking glass, then pour the Virgil's root beer all over and serve with a straw. As simple as it gets, but oh so satisfying!

- **Hot Fudge Sundaes.** I make these with organic Soy Delicious ice cream, Ah!laska's organic chocolate syrup, and soy whipped cream. Choose your favorite cut-up fruits for toppings. We love coconut, kiwi, strawberries, bananas, and raspberries.

- **Sunspire Organic Chocolate.** I'm especially addicted to the dark-chocolate-covered blueberries and dark-chocolate-covered almonds (sunspire.com).

- **Kettle Chips.** I love the sea salt and vinegar flavor (kettlefoods.com).

- **Fried Veggies.** Roll sliced zucchini, leeks, eggplant, and tomatoes in a homemade batter of organic breadcrumbs, an egg, sea salt, pepper, and oregano (to taste) and fry in organic safflower or canola oil until brown and crispy. You won't believe how delicious they are!

Greener Additives Guide

I've already told you the top food additives to avoid. But there are a million more popping up on ingredient lists every day. Fortunately, CSPI researchers say that most are harmless. But if you see an ingredient you're not familiar with, skip the snack or check here to see how it rates. (All info courtesy of the CSPI.)

Safe

- Alginate
- Alpha-tocopherol (Vitamin E)
- Ascorbic acid (Vitamin C)
- Beta-carotene
- Calcium propionate
- Calcium stearoyl lactylate
- Carrageenan

- Casein
- Citric acid
- Diacylglycerol
- EDTA
- Erythorbic acid
- Ferrous gluconate
- Fumaric acid
- Gelatin
- Glycerin (glycerol)
- Gums: arabic, furcellaran, ghatti, guar, karaya, locust bean, xanthan
- Lactic acid
- Lecithin
- Mono- and diglycerides
- Neotame
- Oligofructose
- Phosphate salts
- Phosphoric acid
- Polysorbate 60, 65, 80
- Potassium sorbate
- Propylene glycol alginate
- Sodium ascorbate
- Sodium benzoate
- Sodium carboxymethylcellulose (CMC)

- Sodium caseinate
- Sodium citrate
- Sodium propionate
- Sodium stearoyl lactylate
- Sorbic acid
- Sorbitan monostearate
- Starch, modified
- Starch
- Sterol esters
- Sucralose
- Thiamin mononitrate
- Triacetin (glycerol triacetate)
- Vanillin, ethyl
- Vanillin
- Vegetable oil

Cut Back

The CSPI says these additives are not toxic, but large amounts may be unsafe or promote bad nutrition.

- Caffeine
- Corn syrup
- Dextrose (corn syrup, glucose)
- High fructose corn syrup

- Hydrogenated starch
- Hydrolysate
- Invert sugar
- Lactitol
- Maltitol
- Mannitol
- Polydextrose
- Salatrim
- Salt
- Sorbitol
- Sugar
- Tagatose

Caution

The CSPI says these additives may pose a risk and need to be better tested. Try to avoid them.

- Artificial colorings: Citrus Red, Red No. 40
- Brominated vegetable Oil (BVO)
- Butylated hydroxyanisole (BHA)
- Butylated hydroxytoluene (BHT)
- Heptyl paraben
- Quinine

Avoid if You're Allergy Prone

These additives can occasionally cause reactions.

- Artificial and natural flavoring
- Artificial coloring: Yellow No. 5
- Beta-carotene
- Caffeine
- Carmine (cochineal)
- Casein
- Gum tragacanth
- HVP (hydrolyzed vegetable protein)
- Lactose
- MSG (monosodium glutamate)
- Mycoprotein
- Quinine
- Sodium bisulfite
- Sulfites
- Sulfur dioxide

A Greener You

Here's how readers like you have greened their snack foods:

I have found that the more I tell myself I want healthy snacks, the more I actually crave them. I generally have a piece of fruit in mid morning to keep my energy up for later in the day.
—Eliza, 24, New York, New York

I try to avoid what I call "fake food" whenever possible—anything with artificial sweeteners, high fructose corn syrup, MSG, most fast food, etc. One thing that seems like kind of a drag in the food industry is that overpriced/high-end brands don't do more to green their products—for example, why doesn't Häagen-Dazs switch to hormone-free or organic milk (like Ben & Jerry's)? Why doesn't Starbucks consistently offer organic milk as an option in all its beverages? My favorite guilt-free indulgence is Dagoba fair trade organic chocolate—especially the mint chocolate bars.
—Jen, 31, Brooklyn, New York

We buy a lot of organic stuff in bulk, from a food co-op, but sometimes I simply can't justify the additional costs of organic, so I now try to buy the things that we eat a lot of, like oats and soymilk for example, in organic form but buy the conventionally grown (and cheaper) kinds of things, like dried fruits, that don't make up such a big part of our diet . It's all about balance. For snacks and sweets I like fresh fruit in season, applesauce and graham crackers, popcorn made on the stovetop, homemade muffins using whole-wheat flour, honey from our own bees, and whatever fruits are plentiful—even pumpkin and squashes pureed make great sweet muffins. Occasionally we'll eat bagels or a stick of low-fat string cheese. I'm lucky that my family wants to eat healthy and understands the need to be frugal as well. I realize it's a battle in many homes. The more effort I give to this endeavor of a simpler, holistic way of life, the more it nurtures my health and soothes my spirit.

—Jan, 54, Johnson City, Tennessee

My wife and I are in our mid to late sixties. We have been vegetarian for twenty-five years and vegan for about ten. And we haven't bought any foods with added sugar or corn syrup for the past thirty years—ever since our daughter, then aged six, was diagnosed as hyperactive because of the excess sugar in her diet. We cut out all sugar and all foods with added sugar, and that solved the problem. Today, we shop locally whenever possible, at our local food co-op and farmers' markets, and try to buy what's in season. The only snack foods we eat are sesame sticks from the co-op, plus organic popcorn we make ourselves and top with nutritional yeast [for vitamin B_{12}].

—Alan, Columbus, Ohio

Chapter 5

A Greener Clean:
Personal-Care Products

Peorle often ask me why they need to worry about their personal-
care products—it's just shampoo and deodorant, right? Most of us
don't give them a second thought. We buy whatever brand is on sale at
the drugstore, and if we do spend more on fancy department store and
designer brands of moisturizers and eye creams, it's because we think
we're getting high-quality ingredients that will help us look better (and
younger!) for longer. But the fact is, whether you spend two dollars or
two hundred dollars, most of the lotions and potions we use every day
are filled with unregulated, toxic chemicals that have a much bigger
impact on our health and our environment than you might think.

Consider this: The average woman uses twelve products containing 168 unique ingredients daily—and 25 percent of us use fifteen
products or more—while the average man uses six products, for a total
of 85 unique ingredients, says the Environmental Working Group, a
nonprofit public health watchdog organization in Washington, D.C. You
might only use a dime-sized dollop of shampoo or a swipe of deodorant
each time, but chances are you're using them every day and will do so
for most of your life. And you're slathering all these products on your

skin, which is the largest organ in your body and capable of absorbing up to 80 percent of everything you put on it.

Personal-care products are designed to penetrate—that's how they can do such a good job of cleaning and moisturizing. Many of these ingredients penetrate all the way down to the cellular level, which may make them effective but also dangerous to our health. Preservatives called parabens, used in a wide variety of creams and cleansers, have been found to accumulate in breast cancer tumors, while a component of fragrance called musk xylene is absorbed by fat. Another class of chemicals used in synthetic fragrances called phthalates (also used in many nail polishes and plastics) showed up in 100 percent of the 289 urine samples analyzed by the U.S. Centers for Disease Control and Prevention in a study published in 2000. The subjects with the highest levels were those who use the most personal-care products—women ages twenty to forty.

Unknown Dangers

What are all those chemicals doing to us when they lurk inside our body? Scientists aren't sure. More than 10,500 ingredients are used in personal-care products, but only 11 percent of those have been reviewed for safety. That means we have no idea if almost 90 percent of what we put on our bodies is toxic or not. The Food and Drug Administration, the government agency that regulates personal-care products, doesn't have the authority to test any products before they hit store shelves and doesn't do any systematic reviews of safety once they're out there. Like most consumers, I was shocked to learn this— when you see a product for sale, you assume it passed some kind of test to ensure it's safe for you to buy. But that's just not the case when it comes to sunscreen, shaving gel, toothpaste, and everything else in your bathroom cabinet.

The few ingredients that have been assessed for safety were mainly studied by the Cosmetic Ingredient Review, a panel of dermatologists, chemists, and other scientists which is funded by the industry's Personal Care Products Council (formerly the Cosmetic, Toiletry and Fragrance Association). Not surprisingly, this panel concludes that ingredients are safe more often than not. Even if the CIR does determine an ingredient is toxic, it doesn't have the authority to require manufacturers to stop using it in their products, so companies are on the honor system to phase out harmful chemicals and find safer alternatives. And the FDA can't force them to clean up their act unless they receive evidence that a product is "harmful as used." That means instead of requiring companies to make safe products in the first place, the government is waiting for us to get sick.

Taking a Toll

What's even scarier is that we're starting to see the adverse effects of this system, as a small but growing number of studies show that absorbing these chemicals may be—surprise, surprise—harmful to our health. Many personal-care products contain chemicals that mimic estrogen and may increase our risk for breast cancer, according to a 2006 evidence review published in the journal *Medical Hypotheses* by researchers at the University of Pittsburgh Cancer Institute. They found that African-American women tend to use more of these personal-care products than women of other races and have a higher incidence of breast cancer at younger ages—those aged twenty to twenty-nine are nearly 50 percent more likely to get breast cancer than white women of the same age. Also disturbing: Baby boys exposed to phthalates while in the womb (probably from products their mothers use) are more likely to show signs of impaired testicular function and other genital abnormalities, according to a 2005 study published in the journal *Environmental Health Perspectives*.

And though studies on the safety of specific products are few and far between, we have plenty of evidence demonstrating that many of the ingredients in those products are known to cause allergies, cancer, and other illnesses or be toxic to the reproductive or neurological systems when applied to animals or used in other forms. According to a 2004 survey by the Environmental Working Group, personal-care products expose one in every thirteen women to likely carcinogens and one in every twenty-four women to chemicals linked to impaired fertility or developmental harm for a baby in the womb.

It's not just our health that is at stake. Every time you take a shower or wash your face, you're sending all the ingredients in your shampoo, soap, and other products down the drain. And when ingredients like phthalates end up in our urine, we flush them down the toilet. All that waste water cycles back into our environment, so scientists are now finding common ingredients from personal-care products contaminating rivers and streams around the world. "Scientists find UV filters from sunscreens, synthetics musks, or detergents in almost every water sample tested," says Christian Daughton, PhD, chief of the Environmental Protection Agency's Environmental Chemistry Branch in Las Vegas, Nevada, an expert on how personal-care products and pharmaceuticals find their way into the environment.

Get a Greener Clean

Here's the good news: It's easier than you think to find safer personal-care products made from plant-based ingredients that work really well. This market has exploded in recent years, as manufacturers respond to consumers learning more about the risks of these products and demanding safer alternatives, and I think that trend will continue. I'm not suggesting you throw out every product in your bathroom cabinet and buy a ton of expensive replacements or start making soap from scratch. I'm also not going to make you settle for a shampoo that doesn't clean your hair, or a shaving gel that clogs up your razor, just because it's the "natural" alternative.

In fact, I'm willing to bet that if you try a green personal-care product or two, you'll find they work just as well, if not better, than the synthetic alternatives. Just like eating a clean diet promotes better health, choosing chemical-free personal-care products will actually make it easier to get the shiny hair and glowing skin for which you've been paying top dollar. You might want to take a tour of your bathroom as you read this chapter, so you can take stock of the products you're currently using. Or refer back here the next time you run out of conditioner or toothpaste. I'll tell you how to choose the healthiest replacements.

Activist Spotlight:
The Campaign for Safe Cosmetics

If you had heard anything about toxins in your personal-care products before you picked up this book, it's probably thanks to the Campaign for Safe Cosmetics, a small coalition of nonprofit environmental health organizations that decided to make the $20 billion a year beauty industry clean up its act. It all started in 2000, when Jane Houlihan, vice president for research at the Environmental Working Group, went to the Rite Aid across the street from her office and started scanning product labels. The U.S. Centers for Disease Control and Prevention had just released a study finding that women ages twenty to forty had the highest levels of phthalates in their bodies, and Houlihan, who had spent her career studying chemical pollution in air, water, and food, wanted to know how women could be exposed to more of these potential reproductive toxins than men. Her shocking discovery: Although most shampoos, body lotions, and nail polishes didn't advertise their phthalate content, when Houlihan's team sent seventy-two popular products to a lab for analysis, more than 70 percent tested positive. The Campaign for Safe Cosmetics was born.

"We had to ask, what else are consumers being exposed to through their cosmetics?" explains Stacy Malkan, one of the campaign's founders and author of *Not Just a Pretty Face: The Ugly Side of the Beauty Industry* (New Society 2007). "We realized there was no central place to look up ingredients and check for potential health effects." Activists and researchers from a coalition of environmental health organizations, including the EWG, Health Care Without Harm, Women's Voices for the Earth, and the Breast Cancer Fund, began the cumbersome, time-consuming process of building the Skin Deep database at www.cosmeticsdatabase.com. This searchable inventory ranks the safety of personal-care products based on how their ingredients match up with the health and safety information found in fifty government and academic databases from around the world. The campaign also created the Compact for Safe Cosmetics and began asking manufacturers to sign their pledge to phase out toxic chemicals and disclose ingredient information. At press time more than six hundred companies have joined, though most "Big Beauty" mainstream brands still refuse. "Our next phase is to begin lobbying the federal government to do more to regulate the beauty industry," says Malkan. I can't emphasize enough how crucial such legislation will be to protecting our health. While the European Union has now banned more than twelve hundred chemicals from use in cosmetics, our own FDA has restricted the use of just nine.

Ingredients to Avoid

The next time you shower, check out the ingredient list on the back of your shampoo. Chances are, it's a list longer than your thumb, and most of the words are completely unpronounceable! Even a lot of the so-called natural companies fill their products with a ton of preservatives, fillers, and dyes. How are you supposed to know what's safe to use? I've consulted with the experts at the Campaign for Safe Cosmetics, the Environmental Health Association of Nova Scotia (a nonprofit doing similar work in Canada), and Teens for Safe Cosmetics (more on them in chapter 6) to put together a list of the fifteen chemicals that appear most often in personal-care products and have the most potential health risks associated with them. I know it's a lot of long words. And while you don't have to eradicate these chemicals from your life (nor would that be possible), becoming familiar with them will help you evaluate the products in your bathroom and sift through ingredient labels the next time you're stocking up at the store.

For each of these potential toxins, I've included a list of products that I suggest you avoid. These lists are derived come from the "Skin Deep" database created and maintained by the Environmental Working Group as part of their work with the Campaign for Safe Cosmetics (and available at cosmeticsdatabase.com). EWG's scientists have evaluated over 27,000 products to date and assigned each one a score that ranges from 0 (low concern) to 10 (higher concern). They develop these scores by using over 50 scientific and government databases to search for evidence that any of the ingredients listed on a product's label could be allergens, carcinogens, reproductive or neurological toxins, endocrine disruptors, or otherwise harmful. They also take into account how much data is available on every ingredient and apply the Precautionary Principle; ingredients with lots of inconclusive data score worse than ingredients with a proven track record of safety. The products I list here are just a sampling of those that have received scores of 7 or higher. They contain the particular ingredient they are listed under, but their score is also due to a combination of other factors such as the other ingredients listed on their label, and the amount of information available on them (you can look each product up at cosmeticsdatabase.com for Skin Deep's full analysis). I include them to illustrate how wide-ranging the use of these potentially toxic ingredients can be (you'll see high-end, designer brands and budget drug store brands). These lists were accurate at press time, but they are not meant to be definitive, and the products may have changed ingredients or even have been discontinued by the time you read this. Unless otherwise noted, the information about each ingredient comes from the Cosmetics Database.

It's important to keep in mind that the personal-care products market changes fast—manufacturers are always coming up with new formulations of chemicals that researchers haven't had a chance to evaluate yet—especially because unbiased scientists often have a hard time finding funding for their research. (You'll notice some of the studies I cite are more than a decade old. I include them because, unfortunately they're the most up-to-date information available, but it certainly underscores how desperately we need more research on this issue.) Often pressure from the media and activists will spur manufacturers to remove one toxin, only to replace it with another you haven't heard of! So to make your shopping trip as simple as possible, I've also included a list of the products I trust the most, which starts on page 115.

1. Animal Fat

Oils extracted from the hides of mink, emu, and other animals are commonly used as conditioning agents in sunscreen, shaving gel, hair spray, and more. Skin Deep notes that mink oil is likely to be contaminated with pesticides and other chemicals, while "aluminum hydrogenated tallow glutamate" (science-speak for rendered beef fat) was named as a known neurotoxin by researchers in a 2006 report published in *The Lancet*.

Products to Avoid

Skin Deep identified one hundred and four products made with animal fat. Here are some products that received the worst overall scores in their respective categories.

- Africa's Best Kids Organics No-Lye Organic Conditioning Relaxer System with ScalpGuard (Kids Regular)
- MD Skincare Moisturizing Dr. Dennis Gross Body Wash
- Magic Shave Platinum Skin Conditioning Shaving Powder with Aloe Vera and Vitamin E
- Donna Karan Cashmere Mist Shampoo
- Banana Boat Waterproof Sunblock UVA & UVB Lotion with Aloe Vera and Vitamin E

2. Butylated Hydroxytoluene (BHT)

BHT is an antioxidant that's added to products to prevent other ingredients from changing color as they age. A 1980 animal study published in the *Journal of Medicinal Chemistry* showed that BHT can cause neurotoxicity at low doses. Other studies suggest reproductive toxicity at higher doses, and research published in the *AMA Archives of Industrial Hygiene and Occupational Medicine* showed that it can cause skin irritation as well. BHT is found in lipsticks, moisturizers, eye makeup, anti-aging treatments, foundations, fragrance, bar soap, shaving products and depilatory creams, deodorants, concealers, sunscreens, facial cleansers, body wash, blush, shampoo, conditioner, acne treatments, body lotions, powder, makeup removers, toothpastes, styling products, exfoliators, and nail treatments.

Products to Avoid

Skin Deep identified 2,318 products with BHT. Here are some of the products that received the worst overall score in their respective categories.

- Avon Anew Ultimate Skin Transforming Cream and Hand and Nail Cream
- Neutrogena Skin Smoothing Body Lotion
- Elizabeth Arden Flawless Finish Radiant Moisture Makeup
- Estée Lauder Daywear Plus Multivitamin Anti-Oxidant Eye Cream
- Dr. Jeannette Graf, MD Microdermabrasion Kit

3. Coal-Tar Colors

This range of chemicals derived from petroleum waste is used to control itching, soften hard, scaly skin, and dye hair. They often show up on product labels as "FD&C" or "D&C" colors. The Environmental

Protection Agency lists coal tar as a known human respiratory toxin. According to the *Green Guide,* international government research has suggested that FD&C Blue No. 1 and FD&C Green No. 3 are carcinogenic, while D&C Red No. 33, FD&C Yellow No. 5, and FD&C Yellow No. 6 have been found to contain impurities that may cause cancer when applied to the skin. The FDA issued a warning to consumers in 1993 about coal tar being a possible cancer risk, though they've failed to ban it in the fifteen years since. But it is banned for use in cosmetics by both the European Union and Canada.

Products to Avoid

Skin Deep identified twenty-seven products made with some type of coal tar color. Here are some of the products that received the worst overall scores in their respective categories.

- Neutrogena T/Gel Shampoos
- Mill Creek Biotene H-24 Dandruff Shampoo
- Baker Cummins X-Seb T Shampoos
- Stiefel Polytar Shampoo
- Psoriasin Multi-Symptom Psoriasis Relief Liquid

4. Diazolidinyl Urea

This antimicrobial preservative can release formaldehyde (see Ingredient to Avoid) and impurities that are linked to cancer and other health problems. DU may also cause endocrine system disruption at high doses, according to a 1990 animal study published in the *Journal of the American College of Toxicology.* It's added to moisturizers, styling products, shampoos and conditioners, anti-aging treatments, facial cleansers, sunscreens and after-sun products, facial moisturizers, foundation, eye makeup, acne treatment, mascara, body washes, deodorants, concealers, exfoliators, powders, body scrubs, bath oils and salts, contact lens solutions, lipsticks, shaving products and depilatory creams, douches, makeup removers, liquid hand soap, nail treatments, pain-relief ointments, and fragrance.

Products to Avoid

Skin Deep identified 2,413 products made with diazolidinyl urea. Here are some of the products that received the worst overall scores in their respective categories.

- Serious Skin Care products
- pH Advantage Acne Treatment, Clarifying Hydrator
- Andre for Men Extra Strength Hair Remover for the Body

5. Diethanolamine (DEA)

DEA is usually added to products to make them foam and is often listed on products as "cocamide DEA" or "lauramide DEA." The National Library of Medicine has found moderate evidence that DEA is toxic to the human immune system and irritating to skin, while the EPA classifies it as a "known human respiratory toxicant." Once your skin absorbs it, DEA is also prone to forming compounds called nitrosamines, which have been shown to cause cancer in lab animals. It's added to shampoos, body wash, bath oils, facial cleansers, liquid hand soap, bar soap, acne treatments, shaving products, body scrubs, foot treatments, deodorant, moisturizer, hair dye, and hair spray.

Products to Avoid

Skin Deep found 718 products containing either diethanolamine, cocamide DEA, or lauramide DEA. Here are some of the products that received the worst overall scores in their respective categories.

- Nexxus Botanoil Botanical Treatment Shampoo
- Redken Extreme Shampoo
- Vitabath Travel Sets
- Cellex-C Betaplex New Complexion Collection
- Revlon High Dimension 10 Minute Permanent Haircolor

6. Formaldehyde

It's used as a disinfectant, germicide, fungicide, and preservative, but the International Agency for Research on Cancer has identified formaldehyde as a known human carcinogen, and numerous government agencies have determined it to be potentially toxic to the human immune, cardiovascular, respiratory, and reproductive systems, usually when inhaled. Though cosmetics companies often claim their products are safe because they contain liquid formaldehyde rather than its gas form, you only have to smell a bottle of nail polish to know that the liquid evaporates into the gas form before it dries, says Cora Roelofs, SCD an environmental health researcher at the University of Massachusetts Lowell, who has studied the health of nail salon workers. Formaldehyde is also used as a component of many chemicals, including one called quaternium-15, which the American Academy of Dermatology says causes more dermatitis complaints than any other preservative. Formaldehyde has been banned or restricted for use in cosmetics by the European Union, Japan, and Canada, but in the

United States you'll still find it added to nail products, hair dyes and gels, deodorants, shampoos, soaps, and shaving creams.

Products to Avoid

Many nail polish companies have now removed formaldehyde from their products, so Skin Deep only identified thirteen products that still list it as an ingredient—though potentially thousands more contain it unlisted as an impurity or component of another chemical. Here are some of the products that received the worst overall scores in their respective categories.

- Perfectone Permanent Color Creme
- Nailtiques Nail Protein Formula
- Free & Clear Shampoo New Improved Formula
- Nail Magic Nail Strengthener and Conditioner

7. Fragrance

When you see this one little word on a product label, know that may be shorthand for hundreds of potentially toxic ingredients that the manufacturer doesn't want to put on the label. The FDA lets personal-care companies classify their fragrance formulas as "trade secrets," which means they aren't required to reveal their contents, or their potential health effects, to anyone. What we do know: Most fragrances contain highly volatile allergens that are a recognized cause of asthma and skin rashes in children and adults, says Samuel S. Epstein, MD, professor emeritus of environmental and occupational medicine at the University of Illinois School of Public Health and chairman of the Cancer Prevention Coalition. A 1986 report by the U.S. House of

Representatives' Committee on Science and Technology found "moderate evidence" that many fragrance formulas contain neurotoxins and that 95 percent of chemicals used in those formulas are synthetic compounds derived from petroleum (see additive 10). And many fragrances contain diethyl and dibutyl phthalates, which have been identified as potential hormone disruptors in animal studies. Fragrances and their components are ubiquitous in almost all personal-care products; even products labeled "fragrance free" can contain masking fragrances or elements of fragrance formulas. Watch for them in moisturizers, shampoos, conditioners, facial treatments and cleansers, body washes, hair dyes, styling gels, and deodorants.

Of course, I recommend skipping any perfume, cologne, body spray, or other fragrance products as well (more details on these in chapter 6). Most are unbelievably toxic and they're a great example of how marketing hype can convince us we need a product just because it's cool or our favorite celebrity wears it. I couldn't believe it when my then eight-year-old son came home from school asking to wear Axe Body Spray! I've had to ban it from the Imus Ranch as well, as many of the boys who come want to wear it and we must avoid anything toxic to create a truly healing environment for them.

Products to Avoid

Skin Deep has identified fragrances as ingredients in 12,671 products. Here are some of the products that received the worst overall scores in their respective categories.

- Frédéric Fekkai Protein Rx Reparative Shampoo
- Clairol Nice 'n Easy Permanent Hair Color
- Clearasil Total Control Gentle Cleansing Wipes

Nanoparticles

About $50 billion worth of consumer goods (from cosmetics to car wax) used nanotechnology in 2006, according to a *Consumer Reports* study, and by 2014, the market is expected to grow to $2.6 trillion. Manufacturers are touting these new nanomaterials, where chemicals are reduced to sizes about one hundred thousand times smaller than the width of a human hair, as the greatest thing since sliced bread because they can penetrate more deeply and work more effectively. But their risks are mostly unknown. When materials are this small, their properties change, so carbon becomes one hundred times stronger than steel—and previously benign ingredients may become toxic, while toxic ingredients can become more active. Preliminary research suggests that some nanoparticles can be toxic to human tissue and cells, causing DNA mutation and even cell death, according to a 2007 analysis by Friends of the Earth, a Campaign for Safe Cosmetics founding organization. It appears from early research that some nanoparticles (such as those in sunscreen) are harmless, but we don't have enough research and experience with them to know what is and isn't safe. Friends of the Earth found nanomaterials in almost every kind of personal care product on the market, including sunscreens, deodorant, soap, toothpaste, anti-wrinkle cream, moisturizer, foundation, face powder, lipstick, blush, eye shadow, nail polish, perfume and after-shave lotion. As always, I recommend staying away from anything that hasn't been proven safe.

Products to Avoid

Nanomaterials go by a variety of names on labels, including "nanosomes," "fullerene (C60 hydroxide)," "microspheres," "buckeyballs." Beware also any ingredients that start with nano. And watch out for products that contain "micronized" ingredients too. True micron-sized particles, such as those used by the mineral makeup lines Jane Iredale and Afterglow Cosmetics, are safe because they're still too large to penetrate the skin. Other companies misleadingly advertise their nano-sized particles as "micronized" now that activists have raised concerns over the safety of nanotech. Skin Deep identified 360 products that appear to contain nanomaterials. Here are some of the products that received the worst overall scores in their respective categories.

- L'Oréal Sublime Glow for Face Daily Moisturizer and Sublime Bronze Tinted Self-Tanning Cream
- Hydrience hair colors
- Revlon Moon Drops Lipsticks
- CVS Medicated Apricot Scrub
- Neutrogena Illuminating Whip Moisturizer SPF 20

9. Parabens

This group of chemicals is widely used as preservatives to inhibit bacteria, yeast, and mold growth in products. But they can act like estrogen in your body, which may alter hormone levels and potentially raise your risk for certain types of cancer; researchers detected minute amounts of parabens in breast tumors from twenty patients in a 2004 study published in the *Journal of Applied Toxicology*. Other research suggests these chemicals may impair fertility, alter development in infants and young children, and cause skin irritations. Parabens are added to moisturizers, shampoos, conditioners, hair styling gels, nail creams, foundations, facial masks, skin creams, deodorants, and baby lotions.

Products to Avoid

Skin Deep identified fifty-three kinds of parabens in more than twenty thousand products. Here are some of the products that received the worst overall scores in their respective categories.

- AHAVA Time Line Age-Defying All Day Moisturizer
- The Body Shop Vitamin C Moisturizer, For Men Face Protector, and Vitamin E Gentle Facial Cleansing Wipes
- Avon Perfect Wear Eyewriter Liquid Eyeliner
- L'Oréal Kids Extra Gentle 2 in 1 Shampoo
- Phytomer Whitening Day Cream

10. Petroleum and Byproducts

Consider the classic jar of Vaseline: Petrochemicals are an inexpensive way to soften and protect skin. Plus, they make creams and gels smoother and lipsticks shiny. Unfortunately, ingredients derived from petroleum can also cause allergic reactions and contain impurities that cause cancer and liver toxicity. As a result they've been banned for use in cosmetics by the European Union. But here in the United States, you'll find them added to a huge number of creams, lotions, styling gels, wax depilatories, concealers, mascaras, eyebrow pencils, eye shadows, liquid powders, lip products, and hair relaxers.

Products to Avoid

These chemicals appear on labels under names such as "petrolatum," "petroleum distillates," "mineral jelly," "petroleum wax," and "2-nitro-p-phenylenediamine." Skin Deep has identified more than sixteen hundred products with these ingredients. Here are some of the products that received the worst overall scores in their respective categories.

- Elizabeth Arden Eight Hour Cream products
- Bain de Soleil Orange Gelée Sunscreens
- Africa's Best Organics Relaxer Systems
- Vaseline Intensive Care Lotions
- Olay Daily Facials Lathering Cloths

11. Phthalates (Dibutyl Phthalate, or DBP; Diethyl Phthalate)

This class of industrial chemicals is used as solvents and plasticizers in personal-care products—dibutyl phthalate is the component that makes most nail polish flexible and chip resistant. But studies show this chemical can be toxic to the human respiratory, neurological, and reproductive systems. "We've had well-documented evidence since 1985 showing that phthalates can induce birth defects, low sperm counts, and other reproductive problems in experimental animals," notes Dr. Samuel Epstein of the Cancer Prevention Coalition. Significantly high levels of phthalates were found in 68 percent of blood samples from young girls who began to develop breasts prematurely (before age eight) according to a 2000 study published in the journal *Environmental Health Perspectives,* while the 2005 study previously mentioned found that baby boys exposed to phthalates while in the womb are more likely to show signs of impaired testicular function and other genital abnormalities. As a result, the European Union has banned DBP from use in cosmetics, and many manufacturers including OPI, Sally Hansen, and Revlon have promised to reformulate their products. But you can still find DBP and other phthalates lurking in some nail products, deodorants, fragrances, hair sprays, gels, and mousses, and lotions.

Products to Avoid

Skin Deep identified 133 products made with either dibutyl phthalate or diethyl phthalate. Thousands more may contain them labeled under the catchall "fragrance." Here are some of the products that received the worst overall scores in their respective categories.

- Barielle 10 Piece Natural Nail Care System
- Nailtiques Nail Protein Formula
- Chanel Précision Lotions
- Royal Secret Spray Concentrate
- Cover Girl NailSlicks Built-In Topcoat Nail Polish

12. Placenta

Manufacturers are making millions selling products made with extracts from cow and human placentas to women seeking antiwrinkle creams and hair relaxers. Often these products market themselves as "all natural," but in fact, they can be incredibly toxic. Placenta products contain estrogen and other hormones at levels that may spur breast growth in toddlers, according to a few recent case studies. It's restricted for use by Canada.

Products to Avoid

Skin Deep has identified placenta in twenty products. Here are some of the products that received the worst overall scores in their respective categories.

- Z. Bigatti Re-storation Enlighten Skin Tone Provider
- Hask Placenta Instant Hair Repair Products
- PureStrength Close Conditioners
- Earth Science Placentagen Eye and Throat Crème
- Golden Sunshine Collagen Peptide Facial Mask

13. Propylene Glycol

This conditioning agent keeps products from melting in high heat or freezing in cold and helps other ingredients penetrate your skin more deeply. But that also means it can alter your skin's structure and allow toxic ingredients to penetrate, possibly reaching your bloodstream. The National Library of Medicine classifies it as a skin irritant, and animal studies suggest it may cause reproductive damage or cell mutations that could lead to cancer. Propylene glycol is added to a huge range of products: shampoos, conditioners, bar soaps, body washes, face cleansers, liquid hand soap, acne treatments, hair dyes, shaving products, moisturizers, makeup removers, toothpastes, sunscreens, self-tanners, perfumes, colognes, deodorants, toners, foundations, bronzers, nail polishes, lip products, eye shadows, eye pencils, and mascaras.

Products to Avoid

Skin Deep has identified 7,102 products with propylene glycol. Here are some of the products that received the worst overall scores in their respective categories.

- Exuviance Skin Healthy Home Resurfacing Peel System
- Olay Regenerist The Regenerating Collection
- Clairol Herbal Essences True Intense Permanent Hair Color

14. Sodium Lauryl Sulfate (SLS)

Several animal studies have found that SLS can cause skin irritation at very low doses. Because its primary function is to help other ingredients penetrate more deeply, experts are concerned that it may alter your skin's structure, making it easier for other toxins to reach your bloodstream, and preliminary research suggests it could have carcinogenic, neurotoxic, and developmentally toxic effects. It may also release a carcinogen known as 1,4-dioxane. Closely related to "sodium laureth sulfate," SLS is found in shampoos, conditioners, bar soaps, body washes, facial cleansers, liquid hand soaps, acne treatments, hair dyes, mascara, shaving products, moisturizers, makeup removers, toothpastes, sunscreens, perfumes, and colognes.

Products to Avoid

Skin Deep has identified more than 2,500 products with some form of SLS. Here are some of the products that received the worst overall scores in their respective categories.

- Skin Success Evertone Fade Creams
- Revlon Frost & Glow Highlighting Kits, ColorSilk Ammonia-Free Permanent Haircolor
- St. Ives Medicated Apricot Scrubs
- Clarins Gentle Foaming Cleanser
- Matrix Biolage Color Care Conditioner

15. Talc

Cosmetic-grade talc is great at absorbing moisture, but it can also be irritating to our respiratory systems. A 1990 evidence review published in the journal *Toxicology Letters* found that several thousand infants per year had died or become seriously ill following accidental inhalation of talc-containing baby powder in the past decade. "Exposing children to this carcinogen is unnecessary and dangerous," says Dr. Samuel Epstein, noting that some research suggests a potential link between the frequent use of talc in the female genital area and ovarian cancer. The same goes for you. Beward of talc in blush, eye shadow, face powder, perfumed powder, baby powder, deodorant, and soap.

Products to Avoid

Skin Deep has identified 2,212 products made with talc. Here are some of the products that received the worst overall scores in their respective categories.

- Revlon Age Defying Makeup and Concealer Compacts, Love Pat Moisturizing Powder, and New Complexion Even Out Makeup

- Sephora All Over Skin Bronzing Powder

- Laura Mercier Shimmer Pressed Powder

- The Body Shop Spa Wisdom Africa Spa Honey Butter, Vitamin E Hand and Nail Treatment, Of a Man Aftershave Balm

- Hard Candy Shaker Body Shimmer

What to Buy

With all the toxic chemicals in personal-care products, it can start to feel like you must be better off never shampooing your hair or moisturizing your skin at all. Don't worry, that's not the case! As we consumers become more educated and vote with our dollars, Big Beauty will start to clean up its act as well and give us healthier options. In the meantime, there are a growing number of socially responsible companies making safer products that work wonders. While I certainly recommend that you avoid the products that scored the worst on Cosmetics Database, including those listed above, you don't have to green every single product in your bathroom. Small changes can make a huge difference. Here are a few general tips:

- **Minimize Your Beauty Routine.** Do you really need a cleanser and a toner, a moisturizer and a separate eye cream? These are personal choices, of course, but cutting a product or·two from your routine (or using something weekly instead of daily) will save you time and money and reduce the number of chemicals coming into contact with your skin.

- **Choose Mild Soaps.** You don't really want to be "squeaky clean"—most soaps strip our skin of healthy, natural oils along with dirt and grease. Gentler formulas may reduce your skin's dryness, so you need fewer moisturizers and other creams to replace the oils you've lost.

- **Pare Down on Powders.** The FDA warns that most face, body, foot, and baby powders may causes lung damage if inhaled regularly; talc and other common ingredients have been linked to cancer. This is one group of products to use sparingly, if at all.

- **Double-Check "Fragrance Free."** You want to avoid fragranced products, which can cause allergies and contain a host of unknown ingredients, but don't buy something that claims to be fragrance free without first checking the fine print, as many contain masking fragrances to give off a neutral odor. If a product is truly fragrance free, the word "fragrance" won't appear anywhere in the ingredient list.

- **Pick Your Most Used Product.** Or top three or five, if you use a lot. "The things you're putting on your body day in, day out are the most crucial ones to green," says the campaign's Stacy Malkan. The spa treatment you get once a year is less of an exposure issue. Products that penetrate the skin (like lotions) are also more potentially hazardous to you than products that wash right off (like most soaps), but remember that those products are washing right down the drain into our environment.

Eco Shopping List

Remember, there are many shades of green—and the personal-care products you use are, well, personal! You might decide you just can't give up the tried-and-true conditioner that tames your curls, but you're ready for greener shower gel. Or maybe you want to green the products you use daily, but keep the bubble bath you use to treat yourself on special occasions. Don't beat yourself up for not being perfect—every small change you make will help reduce your exposure and the amount of chemicals washing down your drain.

To help you choose what's best for you, I've culled a list of the cleanest products from the Skin Deep database. These products received a perfect score on their safety scale of 0 to 10, based on scientific data from more than fifty international government and academic databases. If no products in the category received a 0, I've given you a few that scored a 1 or 2, also considered low risk; I've noted their Skin Deep score in parentheses after the product name. The Skin Deep database is the best tool currently available to consumers to help us spot problem products and find safer alternatives. But keep in mind, no computer scoring system is perfect. One drawback of Skin Deep is that it can only evaluate the chemicals manufacturers admit to using. Many mainstream beauty brands list only a product's "active ingredients" on the label, so you have no idea what else you're getting. When you're shopping, it's a good rule of thumb to look for companies that promise to disclose all their ingredients—they'll probably be greener by default because they have nothing to hide. Another issue is that so many of the 10,500 ingredients used in personal-care products have never been assessed for safety. When the computer searches for health hazards on an ingredient, it might not find any—but that's because none have been reported, not because we know for sure that none exist.

Of course, it would be impossible for the Skin Deep team or myself to assess the 90 percent of ingredients that still need safety reviews—that's why we need the government and the beauty industry to do their jobs. But to give you a few more options of trustworthy green brands, I'm also including my own personal favorites—the products I choose for my husband, my son, the kids who visit the Imus Ranch, and myself. Some of these are listed on Skin Deep (scoring a 2 or better), some are from smaller companies that I know and trust (although they haven't been rated yet), and some are my own compromise products because I just haven't found a green alternative that works as well. I've tried to include products that are available online and in most major drugstores, department stores, and health food stores.

Hair

Skin Deep Safest Products

- **Shampoo.** Frequent Use (Revlon.com); Korres Aloe and Soapwort Shampoo (korres.com)

- **Conditioner.** Aubrey Organics Certified Organic Jojoba Oil or Rosa Mosqueta Rose Hip Seed Oil (Aubrey-organics.com); Carol's Daughter Hair Oils (carols daughter.com)

My Favorites

- **Shampoo.** Avalon Organics Shampoo (avalonorganics .com); Aubrey Organics Natural Baby and Kids Shampoo; Giovanni Positron Magnetic Energizing Shampoo (giovannicosmetics.com); John Masters Organics Shampoos (johnmasters.com)

- **Conditioner.** Avalon Organics Hair, Bath, and Body
  Conditioner; Dr. Hauschka Skin Care Neem Hair
  Lotion (drhauschka.com); John Masters Organics
  Lavender and Avocado Intensive Conditioner.

Bath

Skin Deep Perfect Score

- **Bar Soap.** Kiss My Face Fragrance Free Pure Olive Oil
  Bar Soap (kissmyface.com); Aubrey Organics Evening
  Primrose and Lavender Skin Care Bar

- **Liquid Hand Soap.** Terressentials Organic Real Soaps
  for Hands (terressentials.com)

- **Body Wash.** Terressentials Organic Fragrance-Free
  Gentle Bath Gel; Korres Shower Gels; Dr. Bronner's
  Natural Bitter Almond Castile Liquid Soap

- **Bubble Bath.** Aubrey Organics Relax-R-Bath (1)

My Favorites

- **Bar Soap.** Aubrey Organics Honeysuckle Rose Vegetal
  Soap Bar; Pangea Organics soaps (pangeaorganics.com)

- **Liquid Soap/Body Wash.** Avalon Organics Liquid Soap

- **Bubble Bath.** Ortiz Mountain Full Moon Rose Petal
  Bath Soak, which is handmade in small batches by
  Arlena Teitelbaum, our chef at the Imus Ranch (call
  800.923.0072); Farmaesthetics Solar Sea Salt Mineral
  Bath (farmaesthetics.com); Spa Technologies Sea Cal
  Bath Powder (spatechnologies.com)

Make It Yourself

Pour two cups of apple cider vinegar into a warm bath and soak. I'm not sure why, but this is incredibly therapeutic and healing to use if you're feeling sad or depressed. I find it lifts my mood after a long day.

Shaving Products

Skin Deep Favorites

- **Aftershave.** Korres Marigold Aftershave Balm; Old Spice High

- **Shaving Cream.** Samantharoma Mostly Hers Smooth Shaving Oil (samantharoma.com); Tom's of Maine Natural Conditioning Shave Cream (tomsofmaine .com; 1)

- **Depilatory.** Serious Skin Care Liquid Laser Pen (beauty.hsn.com;1)

My Favorites

I never use depilatories or other chemical forms of hair removal. Instead I just shave with my organic shower gel or soap. If you have dry skin, try using an organic hair conditioner as shaving gel—it will moisturize your skin much better than most of the conventional products out there.

Oral Care

Beware of mouthwash and other oral-care products that contain more than 25 percent alcohol—when used regularly, they can contribute to cancers of the mouth, tongue, and throat, says the Environmental

Health Association of Nova Scotia. It's also important to avoid fluoride, which is completely toxic and linked to bone cancer.

Skin Deep Favorites

- **Toothpaste.** Thursday Plantation Tea Tree Toothpaste (thursdayplantation.com); Tom's of Maine Natural Baking Soda Toothpaste (1)

- **Mouthwash.** Jason Natural Cosmetics Organic Tea Tree Oil (jason-natural.com); Weleda Mouthwash (weleda.com; 1); Tom's of Maine mouthwashes (1)

- **Whitening.** Tom's of Maine Whitening Toothpastes (1)

My Favorites

- **My Toothpastes.** Jason Organics PowerSmile Toothpaste (no fluoride); Young Living Dentarome toothpaste (youngliving.us)

- **Wyatt's Toothpaste.** Young Living KidScents Toothpaste

- **Mouthwash.** Thieves Fresh Essence Plus Mouthwash (youngliving.us)

Make It Yourself

Mix a dab of baking soda with a few drops of hydrogen peroxide to make your own nontoxic toothpaste. I do this once or twice a week and find it really helps balance the bacteria levels in my mouth and keeps my teeth a natural white. So many of the chemical whiteners make people's teeth so white they clash with their skin tone.

Deodorant

Deodorant is one area the natural products market hasn't nailed yet—that crystal rock from the 1970s just never really worked for me! I don't love using Sure, because although Skin Deep gives it a perfect score, it also calculates there to be an 97 percent "data gap," meaning most of the ingredients have never been studied for safety. But this is one of those compromise products. I find the Avalon Organics or Erbaviva products work well enough day to day, but when I have to give a speech or do something else where I need something stronger to stay sweat free, I reach for the Sure.

Skin Deep Favorites

- Crystal Body Deodorant Spray (thecrystal.com)
- DermaDoctor Total Nonscents Antiperspirants (dermadoctor.com)
- Avalon Organics Peppermint Roll-On Deodorant (Peppermint)
- Sure Invisible Solid Antiperspirant and Deodorant, Unscented (suredeodorant.com)

My Favorites

- Avalon Organics Rosemary Roll-On Deodorant
- Erbaviva Organic Deodorants (erbaviva.com)
- Sure Invisible Solid Antiperspirant and Deodorant, Unscented

Body

Skin Deep Favorites

- **Moisturizers.** L'Occitane 100% Pure Shea Butter (loccitane.com); Organic Essence Lotions to Go (organic-essence.com); Terressentials 100% Organic Body Cremes

- **Body Firming Lotions.** Aroma 1 Nicci Firm and Tone Seaweed Body Treatment (aroma1.com); Earth Mama Body Butter (earthmamaangelbaby.com)

- **Hand Cream.** Barielle Professional Protective Hand Cream (barielle.com); Burt's Bees Hand Salve (burtsbees.com; 1)

- **Body Oil.** Pangea Organics Pyrenees Lavender with Cardomom Massage and Body Oil; Walgreens Sweet Oil (walgreens.com); Terressentials 100% Organic Body Oils; Pharmacopia Body Oils (pharmacopia.net)

My Favorites

- **Moisturizers.** Aubrey Organics Rosa Mosqueta Rose Hip Moisturizing Cream; Dr. Hauschka Skin Care Quince Body Moisturizer; John Masters Organics Blood Orange and Vanilla Body Milk; Susan Ciminelli Marine Lotion and Sensitive Skin Anti-Aging Cream (susanciminelli.com)

- **Hand Cream.** Desert Essence Organics Coconut Hand and Body Lotion

Lips

Skin Deep Favorites

- Badger Lip and Body Balms (badgerbalm.com)
- Perfect Organics Shea Butter Lip Balm (perfectorganics .com)
- Weleda Everon Lip Balm
- Burt's Bees Beeswax Lip Balms (1)

My Favorite

- Dr. Hauschka Skin Care Lip Care Stick

Eyes

Skin Deep Favorites

- **Eye Cream.** Cosmesis Fine Line-Less (4derm.com); Professional Solutions DCX Dark Circle Under Eye Serum (4derm.com); Garden of Eve Skin Care Rejuvenating Eye Crème (garden-of-eve.com); Cellex-C Enhancer GLA Eye Balm (cellex-c.com)
- **Eye Makeup Remover.** Andrea EyeQ's Eye MakeUp Remover Pads (eurobeautysupply.com); Korres Jasmine Eye Make-Up Removal Lotion; Bioelements Makeup Dissolver (bioelements.com)
- **Eye Drops.** Optics Laboratory MiniDrops Eye Therapy (opticslab.com); Tears Naturale PM Lubricant Eye Ointments (tearsnaturale.com); Opti-Free Express Rewetting Drops (alcon.com; 1); ReNu Rewetting Drops

(bausch.com; 1); Visine for Contacts Lubricating and Rewetting Drops (pfizerch.com; 1)

My Favorites

- **Eye Cream.** Susan Ciminelli Eye Cream; Kimberly Sayer of London Cellular Extract Eye Lift Gel (kimberlysayer.com)

- **Eye Makeup Remover.** Dr. Hauschka Skin Care Cleansing Milk

Make It Yourself

Blend 1 tablespoon castor oil, 1 tablespoon light olive oil, and 1 teaspoon vegetable oil (safflower, sunflower, etc.) to make a gentle yet effective eye makeup remover.

Sun Care

Although it's essential to wear sunscreen daily to protect your skin from sun damage and cancer, finding a truly nontoxic sunscreen is easier said than done. In addition to the host of chemicals described in Ingredients to Avoid, most contain benzophenone (also listed as oxybenzone), and octinoxate, which studies show can mimic estrogen and cause allergic reactions and cell mutations that could lead to cancer because they easily penetrate the skin. And, according to a 2007 Environmental Working Group report, 84 percent of sunscreens offer inadequate protection from the sun (no matter what they claim on the label!) or contain toxic ingredients. Your safer bet is a sunblock containing zinc oxide or titanium oxide because these minerals aren't absorbed. Instead they lie on top of your skin, reflecting UV rays before they cause damage. As a result, many mineral sunblocks are very opaque, sometimes giving you that white-nosed lifeguard effect.

Skin Deep Favorites

- **Sunscreens.** Badger SPF 15 or SPF 30 (1); California Baby Everyday/Year-Round SPF 30+ Sunscreen Lotion (californiababy.com; 1); Keys Solar Rx Sunblock (keys-soap.com; 1)

- **After-sun Care.** Korres Yoghurt Cooling After Sun Face and Body Cream Gel; Lily of the Desert Aloe Vera Gelly (lilyofthedesert.com; 1)

My Favorites

- **Children's Sunscreen.** Aubrey Organics Natural Sun SPF 25 Green Tea Protective Sunscreen

- **My Sunscreen.** Aubrey Organics Saving Face SPF 10 Sunscreen Protection Spray and Natural Sun SPF 25

Face

Skin Deep Favorites

- **Facial Cleanser.** See the Dawn cleanser (seethedawn .com); Albolene Cleansers (albolenecleanser.com); Susan Ciminelli Toning Formula with Peppermint, Rosemary and Thyme; Cellex-C Fresh Complexion Foaming Gel

- **Mask.** Sevi Vegan Cosmetics Clay Masks (sevicosmetics .com); Fresh Sugar Face Polish (fresh.com); Korres

Thyme Honey Moisturizing and Revitalising Mask; Cosmic Tree Essential Mask (cosmictree.ca)

- **Toner.** La Roche–Posay Thermal Spring Water (laroche-posay.com); Arbonne Clear Advantage Refining Toner (arbonne.com); Dr. Brandt Lineless Tone(drbrandt skincare.com)

- **Acne Treatment.** Thursday Plantation Tea Tree Face Wash for Acne; Desert Essence 100% Pure Australian Tea Tree Oil; Arbonne Clear Advantage Acne Lotion; Pond's Clear Solutions Clear Pore Strips (ponds.com)

- **Facial Moisturizer.** Susan Ciminelli Sensitive Skin Anti-Aging Cream, Oil Control Formula, and Super Hydrating Cream; Professional Solutions 100% Pure Hyaluronic Acid Moisturizer (dermatologistskincare .com); Dr. Hauschka Skin Care Rhythmic Conditioner, Sensitive

- **Anti-Aging Treatment.** Susan Ciminelli Seawater; Garden of Eve Skin Care Wise Woman Emollient, No Scent

My Favorites.

- **Facial Cleanser.** Farmaesthetics Facial Cleanser with Lavender; Tracie Martyn Amla Purifying Cleanser (traciemartyn.com)

- **Mask.** MyChelle Blueberry Antioxidant Mask (mychelleusa.com); Susan Ciminelli Sea Clay Mask; Arlena Teitelbaum's Moroccan Red Clay and French Green Clay Masks

- **Toner.** Arlena Teitelbaum's Ortiz Mountain Rose Water and Ortiz Mountain Lemongrass Spray

- **Acne Treatment.** Susan Ciminielli Sea Clay Mask is a great nighttime spot treatment; Thieves Fresh Essence Plus Mouthwash or even plain old hydrogen peroxide dabbed on a cotton swab also works wonders

- **Facial Moisturizer.** Jane Iredale Pommisst (janeiredale .com); Kimberly Sayer of London Anti-Oxidant Daily Moisturizing Cream SPF 25

- **Anti-Aging Treatment.** Tracie Martyn Enzyme Exfoliant and Firming Serum; Spa Technologies Oxygenated Renewal Complex

Make It Yourself

- Grind up a half cup of organic almonds in your coffee grinder, then mix with a half cup of plain soy yogurt for a great facial scrub

- Mix one avocado and a half cup of Vegenaise or Spectrum organic mayonnaise and leave on your face for ten minutes for a moisturizing face mask

Body Powder

Skin Deep Favorites

- NutriBiotic Body and Foot Powder (nutribiotic.com)
- Cosmic Tree Essentials Aromatic Body Powders

My Favorites

- Farmaesthetics High Cotton Body Dust (I put it in my shoes and on my feet!)
- Cornstarch, arrowroot, or baking soda from your kitchen are also highly effective

Insect Repellant

Skin Deep Favorite

- All Terrain Herbal Armor Insect Repellant (allterrainco .com; 2)

My Favorite

I make my own bug spray by putting thirty to fifty drops of Young Living's Purification essential oil into a 16-ounce spray bottle filled with distilled water. It's less expensive, better smelling, and more effective than any store-bought product I've tried. The kids at the ranch love it so much that I make little kits for them to take home with them. One boy told me that he always had asthma attacks at football practice because the coach sprayed the entire team down with toxic DEET—he tried my bug spray and felt so much better, he took home enough for the whole team!

Toxic Tampons?

While we're on the subject of personal-care products, it doesn't get much more personal than the products you use during your period. Most pads and tampons on the market are made with synthetic plastics and rayon, which don't breathe well and have very toxic manufacturing processes. Cotton products are chlorine bleached to make them white. A recent report by the FDA found that seven major brands of tampons contain detectable levels of these chemicals, which store in our body fat and have been linked to cancer, endometriosis, and immune system depression. While your exposure to dioxins per tampon is certainly small, the EPA says that no amount of dioxin exposure is safe for humans— and most women use as many as eleven thousand tampons during their lifetime.

Safe Switch: If you can, use pads instead of tampons and look for those made from natural, nonplastic materials. Another option is a reusable, natural gum rubber cup such as the Keeper (also available in medical grade silicone, if you have latex allergies). You insert the cup inside your vagina during your period, where it collects your menstrual flow—though many women find having to empty and rinse the cup a little too work intensive! If you do need or prefer tampons, look for 100-percent certified organic cotton tampons, which should be dioxin free. I like Natracare, a line started by concerned mom and environmentalist Susie Hewson (www.natracare .com). "We don't use any chlorine-bleached ingredients, perfumes, or plastics," she says. "Our tampons are certified organic, 100-percent cotton and our biodegradable pads are made from GMO-free starch film and pulp from small, sustainably managed forests."

Whatever else you do, stay away from douching products. There's no medical reason to douche, as your vagina will self-cleanse naturally. And it may be quite dangerous: Douching can disrupt your natural pH balance, and Dr. Samuel Epstein of the Cancer Prevention Coalition reports that women who douche more than once a week experienced a fourfold increase in their risk for cervical cancer.

Green Your Personal-Care Paper

Like tampons and pads, most of paper products are chlorine bleached, releasing tons of toxic chemicals into the environment, which puts our health at risk as well. The solution is easier than you might think: If every American household replaced just one box of virgin fiber facial tissues and one roll of virgin fiber toilet paper with 100-percent recycled ones, we could save 586,900 trees, says the Natural Resources Defense Council, an environmental watchdog and research organization in Washington, D.C. They advise looking for paper products that are made from "100 percent recycled" and "40 percent postconsumer" (or better) fibers and labeled either TCF ("totally chlorine free") or PCF ("processed chlorine free"). Below are the most and least eco-friendly options on the market, as recommended by the NRDC.

Toilet Paper and Tissues to Buy
- 365 (Whole Foods)
- Ambiance
- April Soft
- Best Value
- Earth First
- Fiesta

- Fluff Out
- Green Forest
- Hankies
- Marcal
- Planet
- Pert
- Seventh Generation
- Softpac

Toilet Paper and Tissues to Avoid

- Charmin
- Cottonelle
- Kleenex
- Puffs
- Scott

A Greener You

Here are the greener personal-care products that readers like you are raving about:

My New Year's resolution was to live more greenly, so I've switched to Forest Green toilet paper, which is made from recycled paper, because really, shouldn't all toilet paper be made from recycled paper? There's no difference in price or quality. But it has been a challenge to find it in the suburbs. I had to try three supermarkets to find it!

—Michelle, 38, Emmaus, Pennsylvania

I've found that my natural shampoo (Big by Lush) lathers up more than any other shampoo I've ever used. I also love the smells and just how good it feels. I never really considered myself a chemical person, but when you think about how much we put on ourselves, it's almost silly. Knowing that I'm taking small steps to be healthier and cleaner makes me feel good. My friend once told me we shouldn't put anything on our bodies we wouldn't stick in our own mouths and digest. It makes sense.

—Jennifer, 25, Houston, Texas

Long before I started getting interested in green products in general, I was already trying to buy mild, natural personal-care products because I have eczema and freakishly sensitive skin. So I've been a big fan of stuff like Aveeno oatmeal bath and Kiss My Face olive oil soap for years. I also buy Tom's of Maine toothpaste because it doesn't have artificial sweeteners. And I love those "glide" types of dental floss, but it turns out that they're coated in that nasty Teflon-like material. I also try to avoid parabens, perfumes, and fragranced products, both for the pthalates and my sensitive skin. I've never understood why so many moisturizers are so heavily fragranced—those kinds of drying ingredients kind of defeat the point!

—Jen, 31, Brooklyn, New York

I used the Keeper for many years. I love it and I love not adding to the waste stream [with tampons and pads]. Although it's very different from the mainstream concept of menstrual products, it is really a lot more sanitary and less messy than pads or tampons.

—Pat, 65, Columbus, Ohio

Chapter 6

Not So Pretty: Makeup

I've decided to devote an entire chapter to cosmetics because I find they are actually among the hardest parts of your life to green. One reason is psychology—we women get very attached to our makeup! Perhaps you have fond memories of playing dress-up with a certain lipstick as a little girl, or the first time you wore mascara to a school dance. Maybe you wear a particular perfume because it reminds you of your mother, or you schedule your weekly manicure because it's a chance to catch up with your best friend. Though they might seem frivolous, beauty rituals are definitely a way we bond with other women, as well as a way we unwind and treat ourselves. Many women I talk to are concerned that going green means giving all that up—or worse, becoming one of those earthy hippie types who don't even shower, let alone paint their nails! Add in all the more practical reasons we wear cosmetics—to look younger, to cover up blemishes, to seem more professional—and it's easy for a product's ingredient list to be the last thing on your mind when you decide to buy it.

But it shouldn't be. Just like the rest of the personal-care-products market, cosmetics are completely unregulated by the FDA. The industry claims to police itself for safety but doesn't do a very good job. In addition to the chemicals I described to you in chapter 5, the products we put on our face, hair, and nails often contain many more ingredients with the potential for equally frightening health consequences. Frankly, it makes me angry that we pay so much money for lipsticks, eye shadows, and other products that are manufactured and marketed solely to women and young girls, yet contain chemicals that have been linked to serious female health issues like breast cancer and reproductive diseases.

Another reason it's so hard to find good green cosmetics is chemistry. "It's easier to make a cream [or a lotion] out of 100 percent natural or organic ingredients than it is to make color cosmetics," explains Kristin Adams, president of Afterglow Cosmetics, a California-based company that was one of the first signers of the Compact for Safe Cosmetics. Adams uses almost exclusively natural and certified organic ingredients in all of her makeup. "When you're trying to create a natural product with pigments and minerals, you find that many of the necessary ingredients contain something questionable." As a result, there are currently fewer options on the market for safe and healthy makeup than there are for many other personal-care products. Companies like Afterglow Cosmetics are working hard, but it's just taking longer to develop the cleanest technology.

And when a company does come up with a new green product that starts to sell well, you can be sure that the mainstream cosmetics companies will hop on that bandwagon, often losing sight of the original environmental health principles in the process. One example of this is the new "mineral makeup" trend. These foundations, blushes, eye shadows, and lipsticks are made from naturally occurring minerals, including zinc oxide, and titanium dioxide (the same ingredients used in the safer sunblocks that turn lifeguards' noses white) and ultramarine (derived from lapis lazuli, a semiprecious stone). "Since these minerals are inert, you don't need to add preservatives like parabens and other toxic ingredients to make the product last," explains Adams. They also provide natural sun block and are less likely to cause allergies than many other kinds of cosmetics, which are chock-full of irritating ingredients.

But that's only if the company making the mineral makeup is really doing what it claims. As sales have skyrocketed (Bare Escentuals mineral makeup products sold on QVC have seen a 217-percent sales increase since 2002, reports the *New York Times*), almost every major beauty company from Neutrogena to Urban Decay has introduced their own mineral makeup line as have many lesser-known labels. The problem is that there's no official definition of the "mineral makeup," so there's nothing to stop these companies from using just a little of the real minerals and filling up the rest of their products with cheap, toxic ingredients like talc, parabens, and petrochemicals.

Of course no beauty company is going to advertise that it's using cheap, potentially toxic ingredients. In fact, they'll often tell you just the opposite. As consumer demand for green products grows, an unfortunate side effect is "greenwashing"—companies that claim to produce sustainable, healthy goods but never really practice what they preach. It's difficult to spot greenwashing. You need to sift through a lot of often hard to find information with a trained eye. And both large and small companies are guilty—sometimes a company will make a few products that meet all my environmental health standards and then several others that just don't measure up. But never fear. I've done a lot of the work for you by talking to activists, scientists, and the cosmetic companies themselves. Remember that becoming an educated consumer and making small changes are what matter most—nobody is saying you need to throw out your entire cosmetics bag or stop performing the beauty rituals you love. Read on and I'll help you understand what to avoid in most mainstream makeup and which products are safe to buy and will keep you beautiful and confident that you are doing right by your health.

Activist Spotlight

Teens for Safe Cosmetics (TFSC)

Marin County, California, has one of the highest rates of cancer in the entire country. Between 1994 and 2002, the county's average breast cancer rate rose by 60 percent. As a result, "our whole community is very active on the issue of cancer prevention. We shop at the farmers' market, eat organic, and try to reduce our exposure to toxins whenever we can," says Jessica Assaf, seventeen, one of TFSC's founders. "We were worrying about what we put in our bodies, but we realized that we really had no idea what we were putting on our bodies every day." The Marin Cancer Project recognized that teenagers are some of the biggest users of cosmetics, and therefore potentially the most at risk, so founder Judi Shils recruited her daughter Erin, Jessica, and their friends to start connecting those dots in 2005. "I've been using thirty products a day since I was twelve, and my nine-year-old sister gets manicures and wears lip gloss," says Jessica. "I was shocked when I learned how little the FDA is doing to make sure those products are safe."

The girls decided to get organized. They gathered teens from every high school in the county to sit down with a group of local scientists and analyze the contents of the beauty products they used the most, then launched a public aware-ness campaign to tell other teenagers about the toxic ingre-dients they found. Then TFSC began targeting the beauty companies themselves, dressing up as beauty queens with sashes that said "Miss Treatment" to protest the fact that OPI had removed toxic chemicals from their nail polishes in

Europe, but not in the United States. In August 2006, the company (along with Revlon, Sally Hansen, and Orly) finally agreed to ditch formaldehyde, toluene, and dibutyl phthalate from their products. "We realized that if one action can make such a huge difference, we need to keep doing that," says Jessica. The group has since protested in San Francisco's Union Square, wearing prom dresses and combat boots and collecting hundreds of signatures on petitions. They've also launched their New York City chapter to bring the fight nationwide and developed their own line of beauty products now available at Whole Foods Market.

One of their biggest victories came in 2005, when TFSC gave compelling testimonies to the California State Senate to help pass SB 484, known as the Safe Cosmetics Act. This groundbreaking piece of legislation makes California the first state in the country to require personal-care product manufacturers to disclose any ingredients that may be carcinogens or reproductive toxins to the state's department of health before they can be sold in stores. The beauty industry lobbied hard against the bill but lost—and at press time similar legislation was pending in Washington and other states. For more information, visit teens4sc.org.

Ingredients to Avoid

In addition to the chemicals I covered in chapter 5, which appear in all kinds of personal care products, including makeup, there are a handful that seem to pop up in cosmetics alone. I suggest you take some time to become familiar with these as well. Knowing what to look for on labels will help you evaluate new cosmetics when you see them in stores. It will also help you understand why some kinds of cosmetics, such as nail polish, fragrance, and hair dye, are more toxic than others. I've also included products that contain each potentially toxic ingredient, according to analysis by the Environmental Working Group in their Skin Deep Database. (Once again, it's important to note that these products are listed here because they received a score of 7 or higher, though they are just a sampling of the products in Skin Deep which scored this way. They contain the particular ingredient they are listed under, but their score is also due to a combination of other factors such as the other ingredients listed on their label, and the amount of information available on them. These lists were accurate at press time, but they are not meant to be definitive, and the products may have changed ingredients or even have been discontinued by the time you read this. See cosmeticsdatabase.com for updates and a product's full analysis.)

Above all, don't let this list terrify you—in addition to telling you what not to buy, I'm also going to tell you what you can buy, and how to use your cosmetics more safely, starting on page 145.

1. Methacrylate Monomers

This liquid acrylic is the building block of most artificial nails. The industry first developed a form of the monomer called methyl methacrylate (MMA), which is so toxic it's one of the few cosmetic ingredients that the FDA has actually restricted. Reports of contact dermatitis and fingernail damage and deformity prompted the FDA to issue widespread recalls of nail products made with 100-percent MMA in the 1970s, and at least thirty states have banned it since. But MMA can still be found in many salons, and unless you study the product's label, you probably won't be able to tell the difference between that and ethyl methacrylate (EMA), the chemical that most brand-name acrylic nail manufacturers (such as OPI and Creative Nail Design) now use instead. The industry claims that EMA is safer because it doesn't dry to be quite as hard as MMA, reducing your risk of fingernail damage. But in terms of other health effects, they're equally toxic. Both can cause skin, eye, and respiratory irritation, according to the Environmental Protection Agency. And both have the potential to cause neurological damage, ranging from headaches and dizziness to memory loss, especially for the workers handling them day in, day out, in salons, says Mark Cullen, MD, director of Occupational and Environmental Medicine at Yale University School of Medicine in New Haven, Connecticut. Their impact on our reproductive health is largely unknown.

Products to Avoid

I strongly recommend that you skip wearing artificial nails altogether— there is no safe alternative, and applying them is hazardous to both your and your manicurist's health.

2. Bismuth Oxychloride

Bismuth oxychloride is a heavy metal added to many mineral makeup lines to give products their pearlescent finish. On the scale of chemicals you need to worry about, "this isn't the worst ingredient out there," says Kristen Adams of Afterglow Cosmetics. "Some women do just fine with it on their skin. But we don't use it because we've found that some women do find it causes itching, breakouts and general irritation." And if you've ever suffered from heavy-metal toxicity (such as mercury or lead poisoning) you're better off skipping it, as Adams reports it can bioemulate and make your heavy metals blood-level tests "go through the roof." You will find it in otherwise-clean product lines, such as Jane

Iredale Mineral Cosmetics, so if you're not sure how you'll react, consult your doctor and do a patch test with a product before using it regularly.

Products to Avoid

Skin Deep identified bismuth oxychloride in 1,540 products. Here are some to avoid even if you're not worried about a skin reaction, because they also contain a host of other potentially toxic ingredients and received a score of 7 to 9 from Skin Deep.

- Revlon Age Defying Makeup and Concealer Compacts
- Revlon Super Lustrous Frost Lipstick and Moon Drops Frost Moisture Frost Lipstick
- Sue Devitt Studio Lipstick
- Mary Kay Creme-to-Powder Foundation

3. Ethyl Acetate

This chemical, which is the ester of ethyl alcohol and acetic acid, acts as a solvent in many nail products, mascaras, tooth-whitening products, and perfumes. But the National Library of Medicine classifies it as a neurotoxin in its Haz-Map occupational health database, and the European Union considers ethyl acetate an occupational hazard at high doses and warns that it's highly flammable and irritating to eyes, skin, and lungs, while its vapors may cause drowsiness and dizziness.

Products to Avoid

Skin Deep identified 248 products containing ethyl acetate. Here are some of the products that received the worst overall scores in their respective categories.

- Barielle 10 Piece Natural Nail Care System

- Nailtiques Nail Protein Formulas

- Sally Hansen Teflon Tuff Products

- OPI Nail Treatments

4. Hydroquinone

This liquid is so toxic that the FDA issued a warning against it in 2006 and is considering a partial ban on skin lightening products that contain it. (Its use is already restricted in Canadian cosmetics.) Why? It is suspected to cause a skin disease called ochronosis, which causes disfiguring blue-black lesions and small black bumps to develop all over your skin. Also, animal studies dating back to the 1920s suggest that hydroquinone can be toxic to the neurological system even at low doses; the EPA classifies it as a known human respiratory toxicant; and the European Union classifies it as a skin irritant and notes that it may also cause cancer. Hydroquinone is most often used in skin lightening products, but it can also be added to other kinds of face creams as well as hair dyes and fragrances.

Products to Avoid

No product containing hydroquinone is considered low risk. Skin Deep identified 105 products, all scoring at moderate or high risk. Here are some of the products that received the worst overall scores in their respective categories.

- Palmer's Skin Success Eventone Fade Creams

- Ambi Skin Discoloration Fade Creams

- Esotérica Fade Creams
- PCA Skin Pigment Control Kits
- philosophy When Lightening Strikes Cream and A Pigment of Your Imagination Serum

5. Lead

You probably don't need me to tell you that lead is toxic—after all, we know now that any amount of lead can cause damage to a child's developing brain, and the government has banned it from gasoline and house paint for years. The EPA defines it as a possible human carcinogen and a known respiratory toxin, while the European Union says it may impair fertility and cause harm to a fetus in the womb and bans it from all cosmetics. But the FDA approves a version of the metal called lead acetate for use in all cosmetics except those used around the eyes, and as a result, it's often added to hair dyes (both salon and home brands), styling products, and dandruff treatments. A 2007 study by the Campaign for Safe Cosmetics found that more than half of thirty-three lipsticks from major department store and drugstore brands contained detectable levels of lead, with one-third of the samples exceeding the FDA's safety limit for lead in candy.

Products to Avoid

Be aware that lead can also appear on product labels as lead salt, lead diacetate, and plumbous acetate, and that none of the lipsticks containing lead listed it on their labels at all—so there may be many more lead-containing cosmetics on the market.

- Youthair Liquid Hair Conditioner and Groomer and Creme

- EBL GreyBan

- Grecian Formula 16 Haircolor Liquid with Conditioner; Grecian Plus Gradual Haircolor Foam; Grecian Formula 16 Haircolor Cream with Conditioner

- Maybelline NY Moisture Extreme Lipstick in Scarlet Shimmer, Midnight Red, and Cocoa Plum

- Cover Girl Incredifull Lipcolor in Maximum Red and Continuous Color Lipstick in Cherry Brandy

- L'Oréal Colour Riche Lipstick in True Red and Classic Wine

- Dior Addict Lipstick in Positive Red

- PeaceKeeper Paint Me Compassionate Lipstick

6. Mercury

We already know that mercury can damage brain function even at low levels, is a potential cause of autism, and can cause changes in the behavior of blood vessel cells that can lead to cardiovascular disease, according to a National Institutes of Health study published in the June 2007 issue of *International Journal of Toxicology*. But while most of the media hype has focused on fish, cosmetics companies have been slipping this heavy metal, usually as thimerosal, its preservative form, into mascaras and eye drops as well. Researchers at the Environmental Working Group warn that if you get a little bit of mascara in your eyes when it clumps or as you wash it off, you may be getting a little dose of mercury as well. Given all the ways we're exposed to mercury that we can't control (food, air, water), it makes no sense to get even the tiniest amount from a product like mascara, which you can easily avoid.

Products to Avoid

Here are the products that Skin Deep identified as containing mercury or thimerosal. But keep in mind, it could also be listed as mercuric oxide, phenyl mercuric acetate, phenyl mercuric benzoate, phenyl mercuric bromide, phenyl mercuric chloride, and phenyl mercuric borate—so there may be many more mercury-laden products out there.

- Paula Dorf Complete Hollywood 6-piece Eye Kit and Cake Mascaras
- BHI Traumeel Ointment
- Similasan Earache Relief and Healthy Relief Eye Drops

7. P-Phenylenediamine

This chemical is a component of many coal tar colors (carcinogens added to hair dyes and other products) and so toxic that even the Personal Care Products Council concedes that "it may cause cancer" because numerous animal studies and lab tests have found it can spur cell mutations and even tumor growth. Additional animal research demonstrates that it can also cause neurological and endocrine damage at moderate to high doses. The EPA considers it a hazardous air pollutant that is also suspected of causing kidney, liver, and respiratory system toxicity, while the National Library of Medicine notes in its Haz-Map occupational health database that it may cause asthma and skin irritation. P-phenylenediamine is added to most permanent hair dyes, as well as some shampoos, hair sprays, and conditioners.

Products to Avoid

Skin Deep identified 707 products containing p-phenylenediamine. Here are some of the worst overall scores in their respective categories.

- Hydrience Crème Moisturizing System, Natural Instincts Hair Color, Loving Care Hair Color Crème, Balsam Lasting Color Hair Color, and Nice 'n Easy Permanent Hair Color

- Dark and Lovely Permanent Hair Color

- Revlon ColorSilk Ammonia-Free Permanent Hair Color and High Dimension Permanent Hair Color

- L'Oréal Preference Hair Color, Couleur Experte Hair Color, Féria Multi-Faceted Shimmering Colour Gel, ColorSpa Moisture Actif Hair Color

- 100% Color Hair Color

- Naturtint Permanent Hair Colorant

8. Toluene

This solvent is added to nail products to help them adhere to your nail and give polish its glossy finish, but according to the European Union and Proposition 65 (an important piece of legislation also known as the California Safe Drinking Water and Toxic Enforcement Act of 1986), toluene can be toxic to the development of babies and young children. The EPA Office of Pollution Prevention and Toxics notes that overexposure to toluene in nail products may cause irritation to eyes and nose, weakness, exhaustion, confusion, dizziness, headaches, dilated pupils, runny eyes, anxiety, muscle fatigue, inability to sleep, skin rashes, and liver and kidney damage. Because of pressure from activists like the Teens for Safe Cosmetics and legislation in the European Union, OPI, Revlon, and other leading nail brands have promised to remove toluene from their products, though they haven't specified a timeline. But the Food and Drug Administration has yet to require companies to do so, and it still appears in many nail products as well as hair dyes.

Products to Avoid

Skin Deep identified more than two thousand products containing some form of toluene. Here are some of the products that received the worst overall scores in their respective categories.

- Nailtiques Nail Protein Formula
- OPI Nail Treatments Nail Envy, Natural Nail Strengthener, and Nail Lacquer (note: At press time OPI had promised to remove toluene from its products)
- Lippmann Collection Nail Lacquer and Ridge Filler Base Coat
- Delux Beauty Nail Polish
- Funky Fingers Nail Polish
- Orly Nail Color

At press time, Skin Deep did not include the popular brand Essie in its listings, but Essie nail polishes purchased from New York–area drugstores did list toluene as an ingredient.

Eco Shopping List

Unfortunately, a lot of these chemicals are impossible to avoid altogether because we're also encountering them in our air, water, food, and other consumer goods. Look at your cosmetics bag as a place where you can reduce or even eliminate some unnecessary additional exposures. The list below gives you the cleanest products from the Skin Deep database, meaning those that scored a 2 or better (denoting low risk) in their scientific analysis (unless no low-risk products were found for a particular category, in which case I've given you the best of the moderate-risk group; I've noted their Skin Deep score in parentheses after the product name). I'm also including all the products I use and love, and (for the teen perspective!) the products that Jessica Assaf, of Teens for Safe Cosmetics, uses and loves too. The extraordinary work Jessica has done has made her a real hero of mine. And she also happens to be a beautiful young woman with fabulous taste—proof that you can go green without sacrificing your personal style. Most of the brands listed here are available in the Whole Body section of Whole Foods Markets and other health stores; many are also in mainstream pharmacies and department stores. Whenever possible I've also included a Web site to help you track them down.

Now, let's go shopping!

Fragrance/Perfume

The vast majority of perfumes, colognes, body sprays, and other fragrances are unbelievably toxic—and worse, we have no idea exactly what's in them, because manufacturers are allowed to use the word "fragrance" on labels to protect trade secrets. Here are some safer options:

Skin Deep Perfect Score

- **For Men.** Dropwise Essentials Aromatic Mister, Divine (dropwise.com); Trillium Organics Aromarolla (Lavender Geranium) (trilliumorganics.com); Cosmic Tree Essentials Aromatic Body Mist, Lemon Tree (1); The Art of Shaving Eau de Toilette, Sandalwood Essential Oil (theartofshaving.com; 2); Aubrey Organics Ginseng Mint Aftershave (2)

- **For Women.** Dropwise Essentials Aromatic Mister: Soothe; Trillium Organics Clementine Clove Aromarolla; Earth Mama Angel Baby Happy Mama Spray (1); Cosmic Tree Essentials Aromatic Body Mist, (1); California Baby Calming Aromatherapy Spritzer (2)

- **Body Spray.** Samantharoma AromaSprays

My Favorite

I mix my own fragrance using Young Living therapeutic-grade essential oils. Patchouli and clove are some of my favorite scents, but you should experiment to find the ones that work best with your own body chemistry.

Jessica's Favorite

Teens for Safe Cosmetics teamed up with the natural and organic personal-care products company EO to create their new "I" perfume from organic jojoba oil, pure essential oils of blood orange, orange, jasmine, grapefruit, lime, sandalwood, and vanilla (eoproducts. com).

Concealer

Look for formulas with lower oil content, as they are less likely to require preservatives like parabens. Remember to follow expiration dates and toss your concealer if it's more than a year old.

Skin Deep Perfect Score

- BioElements Power Concealer with Maribright Complex

My Favorite

- Jane Iredale Disappear Camouflage Cream

Jessica's Favorite

- Jane Iredale Disappear Camouflage Cream in medium light. "Not only does it cover up any breakouts, it treats blemishes with essential oils."

Foundation

If this is a product you use daily, it's an important one to green. Because they're worn so frequently and designed to stay on your face for many hours, foundations are the third leading cause of contact dermatitis (doctor-speak for skin rashes) among cosmetics users, according to the Environmental Health Association of Nova Scotia. Be sure to throw out any foundations that are past their expiration date or more than a year old.

Skin Deep Perfect Score

- Purepressed Pressed Minerals Foundations (from Web site)
- Jane Iredale Pressed Foundation, Liquid Mineral Foundation (1)
- Afterglow Cosmetics Organic Mineral Foundation (after glowcosmetics.com; 1)

My Favorite

- Jane Iredale Pressed Foundation

Jessica's Favorite

- Ecco Bella FlowerColor Natural Liquid Foundation (ecobella.com). "The ingredients are completely natural and it blends in with my skin."

Blush

The number-one ingredient to avoid in blush is talc, especially if you use a loose powder formula and apply it with a big brush, which releases lots of dust particles into the air you're breathing. Toss any blushes that are past their expiration date or more than two years old.

Skin Deep Perfect Score

- BioElements Balanced Blush

My Favorites

- Jane Iredale PurePressed Blush
- Dr. Hauschka Rouge Powder

Jessica's Favorites

- Jane Iredale PurePressed Blush in Cotton Candy—"It looks natural with a little shimmer"
- Jane Iredale 24-karat gold dust

Note: Skip these if you have metal allergies—while the PurePressed Blush original formula scored a 1 in Skin Deep, the newer version has been downgraded to a 3 because the company added 24-karat gold leaf for shimmer. 24-karat gold dust scores a 2.

Skin Lightener

Avoid any skin lightening product that contains the toxin hydroquinone. To be on the safe side, try using concealer and foundation to even out your skin tone instead. But if you do use a lightener, here are some low-risk products to try.

Skin Deep Perfect Score

- Cellex-C Fade Away Serum Skin Lightening
- Earth Science Ginsium-C Skin Lightening/Age Spot Creme (mothernature.com; 2)

Self-Tanner

Sunless tanners seem like a great way to get glowing skin and avoid the sun's harmful rays. Unfortunately, most are packed with synthetic dyes, fragrances, parabens, oxybenzone (a potential hormone mimic also found in most sunscreens), and a possible carcinogen called 1,4-dioxane that is banned in Canada. Jessica and I recommend sticking to a safe bronzer if you want glowing skin (see below for options), as it doesn't penetrate as deeply into your skin. But if you do decide to fake bake, here is a safer option.

Skin Deep Perfect Score

- philosophy The Healthy Tan (philosophy.com; 3)

Bronzer/Highlighting Powder

As with blush and other powder products, avoid talc-based formulas and toss anything past its expiration date or more than two years old, unless it's a pure mineral formula (inert minerals do not degrade).

Skin Deep Perfect Score

- BioElements Healthy Glow Face Tint
- Larenim Gooddess Glo Bronzers (larenim.com; 1)

- Afterglow Cosmetics Glow Bronzers (1)
- Jane Iredale Brush-Me Bronze (1)

My Favorite

- Dr. Hauschka Bronzing Powder and Translucent Bronze Concentrate (a liquid you can mix with your moisturizer or sunscreen)

Jessica's Favorite

- Jane Iredale So-Bronze 1. "It gives my skin a natural-looking tan."

Lips

Most women ingest more than four pounds of lipstick during their lifetimes, says the Environmental Health Association of Nova Scotia, creating a direct route of exposure for toxins.

Skin Deep Perfect Score

- **Lipsticks.** Canary Cosmetics Mineral Makeup Lip Color (canarycosmetics.com; 1); PeaceKeeper Lip Paints (iama peacekeeper.com; 1); Afterglow Cosmetics Lipsticks (1)
- **Lip Liners.** Alchemy of Colour Mineral Cosmetics Lip Liner (alchemistsapprentice.com; 1); Afterglow Cosmetics Pencil Lip Liner (1); Jane Iredale Lip Pencil (1)

My Favorite

- Dr. Hauschka Lipstick Novum

Jessica's Favorite

- Jane Iredale PureMoist LipShere in Babe. "All of her lipsticks moisturize your lips and stay on for hours."

Lip Gloss

You should throw out lipsticks and glosses after one year. Avoid petroleum-based formulas, which aren't eco-friendly and can actually dry out your lips, although they feel moisturizing at first, says Kristen Adams.

Skin Deep Perfect Score

- Alchemy of Colour Lip Gloss
- Nutra Luxe MD Luscious Lips Lip Plumper (nutraluxe mddirect.com; (1)
- Burt's Bees Fruit-Flavored Lip Gloss (1)
- Afterglow Cosmetics Natural Lip Gloss (1)

My Favorite

- Dr. Hauschka Novum LipGloss

Jessica's Favorite

- Alba TerraGloss in Dawn (albabotanica.com). "I love the color and it smells amazing."

Eyeliner

You should replace your eye makeup every three to four months, as infection-causing bacteria can build up inside.

Skin Deep Perfect Score

- Larénim Eye Liner (1)
- Afterglow Cosmetics Powder Eye Liner (1)
- Jane Iredale Liquid Eye Liner and Eye Pencil (1)

Jessica's Favorite

- Jane Iredale Eye Pencil in Basic Black. "Smudges really well for smoky eyes."

Eye Shadow

Avoid talc-based products; replace your eye shadows every three to four months and clean brushes and swab applicators frequently to avoid infection-causing bacteria.

Skin Deep Perfect Score

- BioElements Seamless Shadows
- Larénim Eye Colour (1)

My Favorite

- Jane Iredale PurePressed Eye Shadow

Jessica's Favorite

- Dr. Hauschka Eyeshadow Solo in Sunglow. "A great basic color that stays on all day."

Mascara

Here are some mercury-free options that also do not contain parabens and other toxins. Be vigilant about replacing your mascara every three to four months to avoid infection.

Skin Deep Perfect Score

- BioElements Multi-Task Mascara Lash Conditioning Formula
- Jane Iredale PureBrow Fix and Mascara (1) and PureLash Lengthening Mascara (2)
- Ecco Bella Botanicals Mascara (2)

My Favorite

- Jane Iredale PureLash Lengthening Mascara

Jessica's Favorite

- Jane Iredale PureLash Lengthening Mascara in Jet Black. "You can apply layers for thick lashes, or you can go light."

Hair Dye

Skip this, if you can: Women who use hair dyes five or more times per year have twice the risk of developing ovarian cancer, according to research by the Harvard School of Public Health and the University of Athens Medical School. Dr. Samuel Epstein of the Cancer Prevention Coalition notes that there is strong evidence that the use of hair dye might account for as much as 20 percent of all non-Hodgkin's lymphoma cases in U.S. women, while a 2004 Yale University study found that people using darker permanent hair-coloring products for more than twenty-five years doubled their risk for the disease. If you do decide to dye, choose lighter shades and semi- or demi-permanent colors (they contain less harsh chemicals), and opt for plant- or henna-based colors that are free of ammonia (which can burn your scalp and eyes), such as those below.

Skin Deep Perfect Score

- Pinaud-Clubman Men's Hair Color, Comb Brown (clubmanonline.com)
- Light Mountain Natural Hair Color and Conditioner (lotuspress.com; 1)
- Rainbow Persian Copper Henna and Persian Red Henna (mothernature.com; 1)

My Favorite

I highlight my blond hair so I can avoid darker dyes, but there is just no good solution here—we need to pressure the hair industry to step up to the plate. John Masters Organics is a New York City salon that uses only ammonia-free herbal and clay based products.

Jessica's Favorite

- Herbaceuticals Naturcolors (naturcolor.com). "There is no 'clean' hair dye, but these are pretty good—plant-based colors with no ammonia."

Hair Styling

Choose pump sprays over aerosol; the droplets are slightly larger, though both can be inhaled deeply into your lungs and transfer chemicals to your bloodstream, according to the Environmental Health Association of Nova Scotia. Lotions and gels are a better choice, though you should avoid mineral-oil-based formulas; in addition to being petroleum based, they attract dust.

Skin Deep Perfect Score

- **Hair Spray.** Jason Natural Cosmetics Earth's Best Hair Detangler (1); Beauty Without Cruelty Hair Sprays (beautywithoutcruelty.com; 1); göt2b In Control Hard-Hold Hairspray (got2b.com; 1)

- **Styling Lotion/Gel.** Kiss My Face Natural Styling Gel; Bumble and Bumble Defrizz (bumbleandbumble.com); Weleda Rosemary Hair Oil

- **Mousse.** Jason Natural Cosmetics All Natural Style and Shape Mousse (2)

My Favorites

- Giovanni Magnetic Attraction Styling Gel and Magnetic Force Styling Wax

- John Masters Organics Dry Hair Nourishment and Defrizzer

Make It Yourself

- **Hair Gel.** Boil two tablespoons of ground flaxseed in $1/3$ cup of water for ten minutes. Let cool and rub through hair; use sparingly.

Hair Relaxers/Straighteners

If you wouldn't pour Drāno on your head, don't use any hair-relaxing product that contains lye, otherwise known as sodium hydroxide. It's the same powerful alkaline chemical used in drain cleaners to dissolve the clumps of hair and other gunk clogging up your pipes. Even at lower doses, lye can dramatically weaken your hair follicles, not to mention irritate your scalp; dry, crack and burn skin; cause irreversible baldness; and make you go blind. Many "no lye" formulas have now been introduced, but they aren't necessarily better—the calcium hydroxide and guanidine carbonate replacing it are still quite caustic and likely to cause skin irritation and hair breakage.

Skin Deep Perfect Score

No hair relaxers score in the low-risk category, but if you must use them, here are some moderate-risk options. Always follow instructions carefully and never leave the product on for longer than the prescribed time—for best results, have it done by a professional at a salon.

- Dark and Lovely No-Lye Conditioning Relaxer System, Super (4)

- gentletreatment   No-Lye   Conditioning   Crème Relaxer (6)

Nail Products

Most major beauty companies promised in 2007 to reformulate their nail products to be free of formaldehyde, toluene, and phthalates—but at press time, we were still waiting. And even with these hazardous chemicals gone, most use acrylic-based formulas that are still likely to cause irritation and other problems. The Environmental Working Group advises that you avoid polishing your nails altogether if you're pregnant or if you have young children who are prone to mouthing your fingers (common when babies are teething!). Otherwise, look for water-based formulas or at least minimize your use by painting your toenails but not your fingernails (especially if you're a nail biter!). Many removers contain acetone, which can cause headaches, dizziness, nausea, and, in the long term, liver and neurological-system damage. Those without are usually still loaded with the always-suspect "fragrance," as well as ethyl acetate, propylene glycol, and other toxins. Always use any kind of nail product in a well-ventilated room.

Skin Deep Perfect Score

- **Nail Polish.** Honeybee Gardens WaterColors Non-Peel-Off Polish (honeybeegardens.com; 2); PeaceKeeper Nail Paint (3, because they're acrylic based and contain isopropyl alcohol—but they are free of toluene, formaldehyde, acetone, and phthalates, and all the profits support women's health advocacy and human rights issues)

- **Cuticle Treatment.** Badger Soothing Shea Butter Cuticle Care; Dr. Hauschka Skin Care Neem Nail Oil Pen; Burt's Bees Lemon Butter Cuticle Creme

- **Polish Remover.** Swabplus Beauty Care Nail Polish Remover/corrector Swabs (swabplus.com; 2)

My Favorites

I never use nail polish of any kind—instead I polish my nails by soaking them in hydrogen peroxide for two minutes once every week or two. This keeps them clean, shiny, and bacteria free.

Jessica's Favorite

- Honeybee Gardens WaterColors Non-Peel-Off in Valentine. "This is the first polish I've found that is completely odorless and still works." Honeybee Gardens also makes an Odorless Nail Polish Remover that is free of both acetone and fragrance and made from a mixture of alcohols and horsetail extract.

Label Lingo

Cosmetics companies have all kinds of tricks up their sleeve to make you think their products are greener and safer than they really are. Beware of these misleading labels that really have no bearing on the safety of a product:

- **Organic.** Almost 50 percent of consumers incorrectly believe that a personal-care product labeled "made with

- organic ingredients" contains only organic ingredients, according to a 2007 survey by the Organic Consumers Association. In reality, there are no federal regulations about how a personal-care product can use the organic label, so most using this term are made up of 70 percent or fewer organic ingredients. Look for products carrying the "USDA Certified Organic" seal instead and double-check that all the ingredients listed say they're organic to be sure you're getting the real deal.

- **Natural.** Don't fall for any product that simply advertises itself as natural—there's no federal regulation on this term, so even products that are 99-percent synthetic chemicals can claim it. Look for companies that fully disclose their ingredient lists and tell you what they're *not* using as well.

- **Hypoallergenic.** For a product to be labeled "hypoallergenic," all a company has to do is avoid using a handful of the most common known allergens. But they can use any number of ingredients that haven't been studied for their allergy-causing potential, and they are not required to test the product (on animals or humans) before it hits store shelves to prove that it won't give you any kind of reaction.

A Greener You

My favorite concealer is Burt's Bees concealer. It's amazing. I tried it out because a friend recommended it—we didn't really mean to be green, but it seemed kind of trendy and fun. I was very surprised to find that I liked it so much better than other concealers I've tried. It feels so light and blends well; it really does feel like it "breathes" more. I wear it every day and it lasts very long.

—Jennifer, 25, Houston, Texas

I've experimented with all the natural nail polishes, and Honeybee Gardens is my hands-down favorite—it's very chip resistant and it blows me away that there's no odor. My boyfriend always used to complain if I did my nails while we were watching TV together, but now he doesn't even notice. The trick is to apply two thin coats. Because it's a water-based formula, the first one might look a little dull, but the second coat will shine as well as regular brands.

—Marian, 27, New York, New York

Chapter 7

Green Your Style: Eco Fashion

Fashion is often the last thing we think about when we decide to start greening our lifestyles. Eating organic food, using toxin-free cleaning products—these are the most obvious changes to make because their impacts on our health and the environment are the most apparent. You feel healthier immediately when you start eating a cleaner diet, and it's the same with cleaning products. As soon as you switch to nontoxic alternatives, you smell and see the difference. When conventional sprays and solvents smell so unbelievably toxic, you don't need to be a chemistry professor to figure out that they probably aren't very good for the earth!

But fashion is a little different. When you put on your favorite worn-in blue jeans or a beautiful new party dress, it's hard to believe clothes that look and feel that good could ever be bad for our health or the planet. That's because all of their impact happens behind the scenes—on farms when the cotton, wool, and other fibers are grown and harvested, in mills where they are dyed and spun into fabric, and in factories where they are sewn into clothes. All we see is the gorgeous, comfy final product, which—unless you know what to look for—doesn't tell you much of anything about how it was produced.

Unfortunately everything happening behind the scenes is taking a major toll on our health and the environment. "The apparel industry has been responsible for some of the worst ecological damage and biggest human rights abuses of all the commercial arts," says Sass Brown, an assistant professor who studies sustainable fashion design at the Fashion Institute of Technology in New York City. Consider these facts:

- Every cotton T-shirt you own required a third of a pound of synthetic fertilizers and pesticides. (Source: The Sierra Club)

- More than 80 percent of dry cleaners in the United States use perchloroethylene ("perc") to clean clothes, a chemical that the Environmental Protection Agency has classified as a possible human carcinogen.

And perhaps most shocking of all: "The average American bought 56.7 new items of clothing and discarded 74 pounds of textiles (including apparel, bedding, and other fabric) in 2005," says Juliet Schor, PhD, a professor of sociology at Boston College and author of *Born to Buy: The Commercialized Child and the New Consumer Culture*. Whether we're a label-loving shopaholic, a dedicated bargain hunter, or something in between, the ecological footprint of our closets is much greater than we think.

I'm going to take you through your wardrobe's entire lifecycle, from production, to consumption, to disposal. When you understand the environmental issues that crop up at each stage of a garment's life, it's easier for you to make informed decisions about what to buy. As we go along I'll be giving you ideas for small changes you can make to reduce the eco footprint of these purchases.

The goal here isn't to swear off shopping but simply to green the way you buy, wear, and discard your clothes. In doing so, you'll cut down on the number of nonsustainable, mass-produced garments you buy (without feeling deprived!) and choose clothes you'll feel good about buying whenever possible. You'll also help the clothes you love last longer and make sure they go on to be useful to others even when you've finished with them. And you don't need to make every change I'm suggesting all at once. Pick the ones that seem the most fun or the easiest to do and go from there.

Activist Spotlight

1% for the Planet

With all the greenwashing out there, what's a surefire way to know if a company is truly dedicated to creating an organic product? If they put their money where their mouth is. That's the simple yet brilliant philosophy behind 1% for the Planet, an alliance of businesses that commit to donating one percent of their sales to environmental organizations worldwide. This enterprise was launched in 2001 by Yvon Chouinard, founder of outdoor clothing company Patagonia, and Craig Mathews, owner of Blue Ribbon Flies, a fishing supply store in West Yellowstone, Montana. "Both Yvon and Craig had been donating one percent of their own sales to environmental causes for years," explains Terry Kellogg, 1% FTP's executive director. "Their feeling was a company can only go so far in terms of making its own practices sustainable. At the end of the day, we have to support the organizations that are working day in, day out to save the planet."

One percent may not sound like much, but the almost six hundred member companies have raised more than $10 million to date. Kellogg is quick to note that 1% FTP "is open to all shades of green." When you see the seal on an item of clothing (or any other product), it's no guarantee that item was sustainably manufactured in any way. "We lend transparency to one particular aspect of a company to help consumers make informed decisions," he says. "But we do find that one percent of sales is such a high bar, the companies willing to take that on often are the ones who are doing other things right across the board." Visit www.onepercentfortheplanet .org for a list of member brands.

Shopping

Fabrics

When you're trying to decide how sustainable a garment is, the first thing you should do is look at the label and find out what it's made from. It's not as simple as choosing a "natural" fiber like cotton and wool over synthetics like polyester—both have major environmental ramifications. The following pages will tell you what you need to know about the most common fabric types. Then see my Eco Shopping List, which begins on page 177, to find companies using the fabrics suggested in each Smart Switch section.

Cotton

Conventional cotton farming, which makes up half of our global textile production, accounts for 25 percent of the insecticides and 11 percent of the pesticides sprayed around the world, according to the Sierra Club and the Better Cotton Initiative, a nonprofit alliance whose members include the World Wildlife Fund and the United Nations Environment Programme. BCI is working to encourage better management practices in cotton. In the United States alone we spray around 84 million pounds of pesticides on approximately 14 million acres of cotton per year, ranking cotton second behind corn in total amount of pesticides sprayed, reports the Center for a New American Dream. These toxic chemicals have been shown to cause a range of human health problems, such as brain and fetal damage, kidney and liver damage, and cancer. "Not surprisingly, farmworkers suffer from more chemical-related illnesses than any other occupational group," notes Dr. Schor.

I'll never forget a certain twelve-year-old boy with leukemia who came to the Imus Ranch one summer from his home in Florida. His family lived next door to cotton fields, and several times a week when the farmers sprayed the crops they were told to shut all their windows and turn off their air-conditioning. It wasn't safe for him to go outside and play in his own backyard! His mother and I both believe that's why he got cancer. Even if you don't live near cotton fields, you could be at risk as these toxins run off into the soil and make their way into our air and water. "Aldicarb, an acutely toxic pesticide [used on cotton] has been found in the drinking water of sixteen states," says Dr. Schor.

Smart Switch: We're a country of jeans and T-shirt wearers, so cotton probably accounts for the majority of your wardrobe. Whenever possible, buy certified organic cotton. This means it has been evaluated by independent third parties and some state agencies to ensure that no synthetic substances were used in the cultivation and harvesting of the fibers. If you buy just one 100-percent organic cotton T-shirt, you can save one-third of a pound of synthetic fertilizers and pesticides—just imagine the impact if we all made such an easy switch! Hemp and linen are also good alternatives to conventional cotton. "Both of these are amazingly sustainable, naturally insect-resistant crops that don't require

pesticides and need minimal processing to be turned into fabric," says
Karen Stewart, co-founder of eco-fashion label Stewart+Brown.

Wool

The conventional harvesting of wool is a toxic process. Sheep are
dunked in a toxic soup of pesticides to kill external parasites, and their
fleece is scoured with petroleum-based detergents. Workers exposed to
these chemical sheep-dips may suffer neurological damage, says the
Sierra Club, and we don't know to what degree these chemicals may
linger once the wool on the sheep becomes the wool in our sweaters.

Smart Switch: Look for certified organic wools, which guarantee
that the animals have been spared from toxic chemical baths. Recycled
wools, especially cashmere, are also becoming more popular—while
they may not have originally come from a sustainable source, by reusing
existing fibers, designers reduce the need for more.

Casual Synthetics (Polyester, Fleece, Acrylic)

Synthetic fabrics like polyester, fleece, and acrylic aren't necessarily
better for the environment. They're made from petroleum, a
nonrenewable, nonbiodegradable resource that pollutes our air and
water, can cause allergic reactions, and often contain impurities that
can cause cancer and liver toxicity (especially for the workers making
the fabrics). Since these fabrics are hard to recycle, most synthetics
end up buried in landfills or burned, a process that releases even more
toxins into our air, soil, and water.

Smart Switch: I prefer to stick with natural fibers—organic cotton, organic or recycled wools, hemp, and linen. They're safer for our
health and the environment, and they breathe better and often last longer than cheap, mass-produced synthetics. If you're shopping for exercise clothes or hiking gear, where synthetics do tend to outperform

natural fabrics, look for those made from recycled fabrics or that can be recycled—Patagonia, for instance, makes fleece and polyester garments from recycled soda bottles, unusable second-quality fabrics, and worn-out garments. Then they invite customers to send in their beat-up jackets, sweatshirts, and base layers to be recycled into new duds.

Dress Fabrics (Rayon and Silk)

Rayon is a cellulose fiber derived from wood pulp, so like paper products, it contributes to deforestation and requires huge amounts of toxic chemicals to process it into a fabric, notes Karen Stewart. "Eco-tech" fabrics such as bamboo silk have begun to crop up as alternatives, but beware of these new so-called green technologies that often sound too good to be true. "Although bamboo is a very sustainable plant and great to use in place of wood [in furniture], it requires very toxic processing to turn it into a fabric," Stewart explains.

Smart Switch: Tencel (also called lyocell) is a wood-pulp-based fabric that requires less toxic processing than rayon—the Sierra Club notes that most of the chemicals used in its production are recyclable and the finished fabric will still biodegrade. Sierra Club also gives silk high marks for sustainability, as it's harvested from the cocoons of silkworms, especially ahimsa silk, which is carefully processed to avoid injuring these delicate insects.

Dyes

No matter what fabric you choose, most clothes—like all textiles—are colored with incredibly toxic dyes. The most common are azodyes, used on both fabrics and leathers. "It's believed to be a carcinogen and has been banned in Europe," notes Dr. Schor. "One study found that 30 percent of German children suffer from textile-related allergies, most of which are triggered by dyes." Formaldehyde, pentachlorophenol, and heavy metals are other common dye ingredients that pose serious health hazards. Meanwhile, most cotton and wools are bleached with chlorine, which contaminates our air and water and releases dioxins, a class of chemicals known to cause cancer and a host of other problems.

Smart Switch: You don't have to sacrifice a colorful wardrobe to stay healthy—just look for fabrics that are colored with vegetable or soy-based dyes. Check that your organic cotton and wools are also labeled "unbleached" or "chlorine free," as the U.S. Department of Agriculture only requires that fabrics labeled organic be produced without the use of most conventional pesticides or synthetic fertilizers—they don't regulate the dyeing process. The Organic Trade Association does ban toxic dyes in their standards for handling and processing textiles, but these guidelines are voluntary, so ask the manufacturer if "organic" applies to the garment's entire production process, from start to finish. See my Eco Shopping List on page 177 for brands using these non-toxic dyes.

Leather vs. Pleather

This is one of the trickiest eco-fashion questions. Leather used for our shoes, bags, and jackets comes from cows raised for beef and dairy, and most of the leather we buy in the United States is imported from developing nations with less stringent environmental regulations for their tanning industries, reports the Food and Agriculture Organization of the United Nations. For example, the tanning industry that sprang up in South India during the 1990s has dangerously polluted local water supplies with the toxic chemicals used to tan and dye hides. And numerous studies show that tanning-industry workers are also exposed to harmful levels of these chemicals, putting them at heightened risk for lung, bladder, kidney, and pancreatic cancers.

On the other hand, most "pleather" on the market is made from polyvinyl chloride (PVC), a petroleum-based plastic that can contain many potential toxins, including lead and phthalates. Workers exposed to it over long periods of time have an increased risk for liver cancer. PVC production is the largest and fastest-growing use of chlorine, accounting for nearly 40 percent of all chlorine used in the United States. Thus its manufacturing process also creates and releases tons of dioxins into our environment. And PVC is far less recyclable than any other plastic.

Smart Switch: You should absolutely avoid any pleather product made from PVC—you'll know it is if it's inexpensive, shiny, and labeled "vinyl." Less toxic pleathers made from polyurethane, polypropylene, or polyethylene are good options for trendy items, like an "it" bag that you know you'll only use for a season or two. But the more sustainable choice is to shop for well-made goods that will last for years, and in my experience, that means leather. I just haven't found a pleather that can stand up to wear and tear on the ranch the way my leather cowboy boots do, nor do I find pleather dress shoes as comfortable as leather heels. The good news is some companies, like Terra Plana (a British company that makes quirky sneakers, whimsical ballet flats, and even pumps) are starting to offer organic or sustainable leather goods made from free-range cattle and treated with vegetable dyes instead of heavy metals. See my Eco Shopping List on page 177 for more shoes.

Wearing

While the sustainability of the clothes you buy is important, their eco footprints don't end as soon as you bring them home from the store and hang them in your closet. "Sixty to eighty percent of a garment's ecological impact occurs after its purchase," says Lynda Grose, a professor of sustainable fashion design at California College of the Arts in San Francisco. Washing and drying accounts for most of this impact. I covered how to green your laundry room in detail in chapter 9 of

Green This! Volume One: Greening Your Cleaning, but here are the main points to remember:

Washing

Most commercial laundry detergents on the market today contain harmful chemicals that can aggravate our respiratory systems and cause serious hormonal dysfunction. I really encourage you to switch to a concentrated natural detergent such as Imus Greening the Cleaning, BioKleen, Ecover, or Seventh Generation's biodegradable, nontoxic laundry liquids. Whatever brand you use, make sure it discloses all its ingredients on the label and is free of petroleum products, phosphates, chlorine, optical brighteners, synthetic toxic fragrances, and dyes.

When you're programming your washing machine, choose the cold or warm cycles, and always rinse on cold. Heating up the water accounts for up to 90 percent of the energy a washer uses, and you really only need the hot cycle to get out the toughest, most oily stains. And wash only full loads, or adjust your machine's water setting—laundry accounts for 22 percent of all the water we use in the home, and using your machine's small-capacity setting can cut the water used in half.

If you're in the market for a new washing machine, look for one with the Energy Star seal, as they use 50 percent less energy than a standard washer, and opt for a front-loading machine. Front-loaders use up to 60 percent less water and about 50 percent less energy than top-loaders. They also spin faster, so your clothes need less time in the dryer.

Hand washing will also save energy and protect your delicate fabrics so clothes last longer. I wash all my cashmere and wool sweaters by putting a dime-sized amount of nontoxic laundry liquid in a stainless steel bucket filled with warm water. Dip your sweater in the bucket a couple of times, then pat it dry with a towel (never wring it out) and hang it on a wooden drying rack. (You don't even need to rinse!)

Removing Stains

Commercial spot removers are highly toxic, containing chemicals like benzene, perchlorethylene, and trichlorethane that contaminate our groundwater and potentially cause cancer. You'll find you can easily live without them. I get most stains out just by soaking soiled clothes in a bucket of warm water and nontoxic laundry liquid for at least half an hour before washing (really tough stains do best if you soak them overnight). Applying a paste of baking soda and water to the stain for an hour before washing works too—for sweat stains, especially on white fabrics, mixing the baking soda with a little lemon juice works really well. Both Ecover and Biokleen make effective stain treatments that are free of toxins.

Softening Fabrics

Traditional fabric softeners and dryer sheets contain fragrance and other toxic ingredients and are absolutely unnecessary. If you find your clothes stiffen up after washing, try adding a tablespoon of white distilled vinegar (preferably organic) to the rinse cycle, or line dry and air tumble for a few minutes in the dryer. Your clothes will come out soft every time.

Drying

Your clothes dryer is the second-largest electricity-consuming appliance in your home (after your fridge). And while it gets the job done fast, it can also wreak havoc on clothes, shrinking, fading, and pilling them so you end up discarding them much sooner. Whenever possible, I advocate air drying your clothes, either on a wooden drying rack or, if you have the space, outdoors on a clothesline.

When you do use your dryer you can make it more energy efficient by keeping its lint screen, vent hood, and exhaust hose free of dust and drying loads back-to-back so the machine can recycle the hot air from the first load. Dry heavy towels and bedding separately from lightweight clothes, which dry faster so you don't need to waste energy drying them for so long. If your machine has a moisture sensor, use it to prevent overdrying.

Ironing

When done properly, ironing can make your clothes look like new and save you from unnecessary washing and dry cleaning. But nothing ruins clothes faster than improper ironing. Fill your iron with purified or distilled water, instead of tap, which contains minerals that may damage the appliance. I never use spray starch, as most commercial formulas contain formaldehyde, a suspected carcinogen, and can irritate the lungs and respiratory system. Instead, I mix my own ironing spray by filling a 32-ounce spray bottle with distilled water, six to eight drops of an essential oil (lemon, lavender, rose, or grapefruit are great choices), and a quarter teaspoon of nontoxic laundry liquid.

Always use the proper temperature setting when you iron. If you iron a delicate fabric at too high a temperature, the fabric will melt and create a sticky mess, ruining both your iron and your outfit! If you're in the market for a new iron, consider a clothes steamer instead—they tend to be much easier to use and gentler on your clothes.

Dry Cleaning

More than 80 percent of U.S. dry cleaners use the chemical perchloroethylene ("perc") to clean clothes. This potential human carcinogen can cause mood and behavioral changes and irritate the eyes, nose, mouth, and throat at low doses (below 100 parts per million). It can cause headaches, dizziness, light-headedness, vomiting, nausea, unconsciousness, and kidney dysfunction at higher doses and is considered immediately dangerous to life and health at 150 parts per million.

Fortunately, several less-toxic dry cleaning options now exist, and you'll see many dry cleaners advertising their "green" or "organic" services, though not all are created equal. The most common method is GreenEarth, a silicone-based solvent that, despite it's natural-sounding name, comes with its own set of health and environmental concerns. A better bet is to ask your cleaner if they use liquid carbon dioxide in high-pressure cleaning machines. A *Consumer Reports* study found this method cleaned clothes even better than the conventional dry cleaning method for about the same price. Some cleaners also offer "wet cleaning," where clothes are washed with plain water in computer-controlled washing machines. And by and large, most clothes that suggest dry cleaning do just fine with hand washing, or even just spot treating.

If you do have a garment cleaned at a conventional dry cleaner, ask that they remove it from its plastic bag before you take it home. Then hang the garment outside for at least an hour to let the perc dissipate before you bring it inside. Air quality analyses of bedrooms have found that ambient air levels of perc skyrocket when people bring their dry cleaning home without airing it out first.

Discarding

The last phase of your clothes' lifecycle is what happens to them after they leave your closet. "Historically, clothing has been a high-priced commodity and as a result, our garments used to live long and varied lives," says Dr. Schor. "When an outfit was no longer appropriate for special occasion wear, it became an everyday dress. Eventually it would be turned into rags or patches in quilts." Admit it—even if you regularly box up old clothes for Goodwill, rather than tossing them straight in the trash, it's probably been a while since you cut up old dresses to make a quilt. And with the EPA reporting that the average American discards an average of seventy-four pounds of textiles each year, it's clear we're sending a good amount of our old clothes, footwear, and accessories to clog up landfills.

Think Quality, Not Quantity

Instead of buying five tank tops for twenty-five dollars and having to replace them three months from now, why not buy one twenty-five-dollar or even fifty-dollar top in a classic cut that is well made enough to last for several years? Disposable fashion seems cheap, but it actually costs us more in the long run than investing in high-quality pieces we truly love and will want to wear longer.

Host a Clothes Swap

When you do clean out your closet, invite your friends to do the same. Then open some wine and try on one another's clothes. The sweater that never suited you might be perfect for your best friend, while the cocktail dress she never got around to wearing could be exactly what you need for an upcoming party. Everyone ends up with new clothes they love—without spending a dime! In London, New York, and other cities, clothes swapping has become so popular, you can also find large-scale swaps happening at hip bars or clubs. Why not organize one for your next school or church fundraiser? They're especially great if you plan a theme like "Back to School," if you have a lot of friends with children around the same age, or host one around the holidays to help people avoid the mall and work through their gift list.

Take a Sewing Class

No, you don't have to turn your old clothes into patchwork quilts—unless you want to!—but mastering basic sewing skills will help you breathe new life into tired outfits, whether you can handle simple tasks like mending holes and sewing on buttons or want to get more creative by updating an old skirt with a new hemline or this season's trim.

Donate to Charity

But choose your cause carefully. Dr. Schor's research shows that only a small fraction of clothes donated or sold to secondhand stores end up truly helping those in need. Really beat-up clothes get sold in bulk to factories that repurpose them for uses like stuffing car seats. Less worn items are often sold to brokers who export clothes to developing countries. The United Nations estimates that more than 500 million kilograms of worn clothing were exported from the United States to the rest of the world in 2004. "The upside to this is poor people in these countries have access to coveted American goods that are often higher quality than what they can get domestically," says Dr. Schor. "But it also puts local clothes makers, often women, out of business. And there's something sad and ironic about the fact that these secondhand American clothes might be bought by the same people who manufactured them in sweatshop factories in the first place."

Dropping clothes off in your neighborhood Goodwill box is certainly better than sending them straight to a landfill. But to ensure your clothes really help those in need, consider delivering them to an organization like Dress for Success, which provides low-income women with clothes for job interviews (www.dressforsuccess.org).

Eco Shopping List

Here's a roundup of sustainable clothing options at every price point. Because eco fashion is so complex, no company on this list is 100-percent green. I've done my best to research their pros and cons so you can make informed choices. I've also tracked down a range of brands, so you have green options whether you're just stocking up on jeans and T-shirts or looking for something a little more unique.

Couture

Armani

I've always loved Armani's beautiful suits, and I became even more enthusiastic about him as a designer when he began introducing more sustainable materials to his collections. He's made a huge effort to increase his use of organic cotton and low-impact fabric dyes, even using eco washes to distress denim in the Armani Jeans collection. Much of his wool is alpaca, sourced from fair-trade projects in Peru and Bolivia, where farmers raise brown-coated alpacas that otherwise would be nearing extinction because the traditional wool manufacturing industry rejects their dark wool. Of course Armani isn't cheap—but if you want a suit that will last a lifetime, he's my designer of choice (armani.com).

Anna Cohen

This Oregon-based designer's "Italian Street Couture" is 75 percent sustainable. She uses local sources to find her organic and recycled fabrics, minimizes packaging, and fits out her studio with recycled furnishings and office supplies. I like that Anna admits to her limitations, such as having to use synthetic buttons and thread and a small portion of processed and dyed materials when eco alternatives aren't available. Anna Cohen is also a member of 1% for the Planet and a great source for sexy halter dresses, graphic tees and tanks, and skinny jeans (annacohen.com).

Beyond Skin

Natalie Dean, the British creator of Beyond Skin, offers handcrafted footwear made to order from cotton-backed polyurethane (in lieu of leather or PVC) and silks. Her styles include slouchy boots as well as darling T-straps, peep-toes, and wedges in a variety of cheerful colors and have been seen on celebrities like Natalie Portman and Heather Mills (beyondskin.co.uk).

Camper

This European shoe company is a fashionista favorite because its designs are comfortable and well made—but also brightly colored and whimsical (often each shoe in a pair will have slightly different details that make you look twice!). Their Wabi shoe is made from a single piece of 100-percent recyclable thermoplastic elastomer (TPE). To further reduce the shoe's eco footprint, Camper cut back to only four industrial production processes in its manufacturing (most shoes require forty processes and use up to sixty components) so they could use minimal materials, machinery, and manpower (camper.com).

Crystalyn Kae

I adore my Monarch black hobo bag—it's chic and vegan! She uses a great mix of vintage fabrics and upholstery-grade fabrics that have been scuffed, then glazed to be as sturdy as leather (crystalnkae.com).

Edun and Loomstate

Both these lines from eco-fashion guru Rogan Gregory are pretty great. He partnered with eco-power couple Bono and Ali Hewson to create Edun, which offers a full range of edgy, modern dresses, graphic tees, sweaters, and other separates, some made with organic cotton and all manufactured in fair-trade factories that Edun works with "on a micro level" in India, Peru, Tunisia, Kenya, Uganda, Lesotho, Mauritius, and Madagascar (edunonline.com). Loomstate features 100-percent organic cotton jeans, chinos, hoodies, and tops for men and women in a range of vegetable-dyed hues (loomstate.org).

Linda Loudermilk

The pioneer of the eco-luxury category, Loudermilk was one of the first to decide that "green clothes no longer have to be ugly, they can be hip, refined, edgy, and compelling." Loudermilk's team works closely with fiber and fabric manufacturers to create green fabrics from soy and other sustainable resources, and she reports, "In my experience, the fashion industry is really starting to pull together to become green." A great source for chic little black dresses, dramatic wraps, and other evening wear (lindaloudermilk.com).

Matt & Nat

I love my turquoise hobo Matt & Nat bag. They're one of only a handful of designers I've found that do great vegan, no-leather handbags without using PVC or other plastics. Instead they use a good quality material with a waxed finish that really looks like leather (mattand nat.com).

Stewart+Brown

Stewart+Brown is one of my favorite sources for organic cotton and sustainable cashmere—their nature-inspired designs and excellent eye for quality make these clothes that you want to curl up and live in. The cashmere (sweaters, tees, and blankets) comes from small-scale nomadic herdsmen in Mongolia. They also work to ensure fair working conditions in all of their factories and donates at least one percent of all sales to the environmental and social welfare causes (stewartbrown. com).

Terra Plana

This British designer makes funky, bright-colored sandals, loafers, sneakers, flats, pumps, and boots for men and women (as well as a great selection of bags and belts) from a variety of eco materials, including chrome-free, vegetable-tanned leather, recycled leather, recycled rubber, and recycled foam. They work closely with their factories to ensure fair working practices and green production to reduce waste and the use of toxins (terraplana.com).

Midrange

American Apparel

American Apparel recycles more than one million pounds of cotton cuttings per year (most companies send this waste to landfills or let it rot in warehouses) and has recently begun to introduce more organic cotton into their lines of brightly colored T-shirts, tank tops, and other knitwear for men, women, children, and pets. I've bought their signature striped knee-high tube socks because they're great to wear under my tall cowboy boots on the ranch, and that retro style is hard to find at most other stores (americanapparel.net).

Eileen Fisher

Eileen Fisher features naturally green linen and silk and is gradually introducing more and more organic cotton to their line of well-cut dresses and separates. The company has also made an effort to use recycled and reclaimed materials in their stores and packaging materials and has agreed to adhere to Social Accountability 8000, an internationally recognized set of workplace standards. Two social-compliance audit firms monitor Eileen Fisher's factories in the United States and China to ensure the SA8000 standards are being met (eileenfisher.com).

Levi's Organic Cotton

I have to applaud the new Levi's Eco line, as it's one of the few places you can get stylish organic cotton jeans at nondesigner prices. In 2005 the company showed a new commitment toward improving garment factory conditions when it began publishing the names and addresses of all its active suppliers on its Web site. This makes it easier for advocacy groups to track workplace conditions through the supply chain (levis.com).

Nau

FIT's Professor Sass Brown gives Nau high marks for both its "accessible price-points and a sustainable business model," as the Oregon-based outdoor clothing company (which also sells jean skirts, hooded sweaters, chinos, and other classic basics for women and men) says their corporate mission is to "demonstrate the highest standards of citizenship in everything we do." As a result, Nau uses an independent, nonprofit auditing organization to ensure its suppliers and manufacturers protect workers and considers the entire life cycle of a garment when designing and manufacturing their eco fabrics (nau.com).

Patagonia

Both Dr. Schor and Professor Brown rate Patagonia as one of the largest green clothing companies out there. You absolutely can't beat them for quality when it comes to hiking, skiing, and other outdoor activity gear, but they're also a great source for casual tops, skirts, and shorts that look smart in the city or the country, and swimsuits, underwear, and socks. They make every effort to green their materials and production processes—even their hiking boots are made with recycled rubber! And of course, their founder Yvon Chouinard is behind the revolutionary 1% FTP (patagonia.com).

Tsonga Shoes

These cute, comfortable leather sandals, mules, clogs, and boots are hand stitched by Zulu craftswomen near the Drakensberg Mountains in South Africa. The fair-trade brand has managed to rejuvenate the economy of the village by creating jobs and community outreach programs that improve quality of life (tsongausa.com).

Ten Thousand Villages

This chain of more than 160 stores is probably the easiest way to find a wide range of fair-trade accessories and gifts, as the company works with more than one hundred villages in thirty countries around the world. Their jewelry collection is always stocked with chunky glass beads, delicate silver earrings, and artistic cuffs, all at very reasonable prices. Also fun for home décor and hostess gifts (tenthousand villages.com).

Bargain

You'll notice that several brands listed in this section aren't what most of us would consider truly green—the Gap, Wal-Mart, and H&M. But considering that there's barely a shopping center in America without an H&M, Gap, Banana Republic, and Old Navy, let alone a Wal-Mart, I understand that most of us are hard-pressed to avoid these stores altogether, especially if you're on a tight budget or in an area with few other shopping options.

The good news is, each of these stores has begun making efforts to green its business practices, and while they may seem small, when huge companies take even a tiny step in the right direction, the benefits can be big. "Ten years from now, we may find that these big box stores' bottom-line focus has undermined the sanctity of organic standards and made the situation worse," says Dr. Schor. "Or we may look back and realize that without big chains getting behind organic, we never would have made so much progress." The bottom line is, it's too soon to tell how this new industrial organic movement will impact the fashion industry. But if you do shop at these stores, use it as an opportunity to send them a message with your dollars—buy from their eco lines and avoid the less green options.

Gap Organic Cotton

In spring 2007, the Gap introduced a line of 100-percent organic cotton men's T-shirts, to be sold in stores nationwide. They've also joined the steering committee of the Better Cotton Initiative, a nonprofit whose other members include the World Wildlife Fund and the United Nations Environment Programme. BCI is working to encourage better management practices in cotton, such as paying fair-trade prices to farmers, reducing diversion of water for irrigation, and going organic whenever possible. Let's hope these T-shirts are the first of many greener practices by the Gap (gap.com).

H&M Organic Cotton

H&M has also joined BCI (Adidas and Ikea are the other retail members) and begun introducing organic cotton into its stores (hm. com).

Maggie's Functional Organic

Most of the affordable camisoles, T-shirts, pants, socks, tights, and baby clothes offered at this innovative online retailer are made in the Fair Trade Zone, a workers' collective in Nicaragua. They use organic cotton and other sustainable materials as well as low-impact dyes. Plus where else can you find organic cotton textured tights? (organicclothes. com).

No Sweat Apparel

This is the first international union-made brand that makes a range of casual wear like no-logo tees, outerwear, jeans, socks, and sneakers (nosweatapparel.com).

Wal-Mart Organic Cotton

Organic cotton yoga gear and other clothing is just one of a host of green initiatives recently introduced by the world's largest private employer. They're also promoting organic food (see chapter 3 for more info), changing to biodegradable corn-based hangers instead of plastic, and stocking compact fluorescent light bulbs. Environmental and social justice organizations are on the fence about if these changes are anything more than window dressing to disguise Wal-Mart's many other problems. But there's no question that Wal-Mart has more influence than any other retailer on the supply chain, so any step in the right direction is better than nothing (walmart.com).

A Greener You

Here's how these chic readers lengthen the life of their wardrobes, without giving up their sense of style:

We all buy too many clothes, too much stuff. Not one person I know can say they couldn't do with a closet purge—almost weekly. Why do we need another black tee, just one more pair of jeans, a new dress to wear to a wedding just because there are two overlapping guests who saw you at the last one? This summer, in fact, I'm going to six weddings, and I've pledged not to buy a dress for a single one. I have plenty of dresses that will work just fine. I once read that French women's closets have air between the hangers. Isn't that a lovely goal?

—Melissa, 30, Brooklyn, New York

My grandmother, my mom, her six sisters, and I get together a few times a year to hold a clothing swap. My mom started it twelve to fifteen years ago. It's such an easy way to refresh your wardrobe and clean our your closet. Over the years it has expanded beyond clothes, shoes, and accessories—sometimes we bring bedding, towels, tablecloths, books, magazines, baby items, and other home stuff. Anything left over that nobody wants to swap is donated to charity for someone else's enjoyment, so we know we saved it from the landfill for a bit longer. The whole day is a lot of fun and some of my most highly complimented outfits have come from my aunts!

Rebecca, 30, Guilford, Connecticut

I've never been particularly fashion conscious, but I do like to look "presentable," as my grandmother used to say. I decided at the beginning of 2007 to try to go this whole year not purchasing anything new in the way of clothing. I have lots and lots of nice things already (too many, actually!) and halfway through the year, am very proud and pleased to be able to say that I've not bought a single new piece of clothing, and don't intend to—I may even continue my experiment for yet another year, we'll see. I make my current wardrobe last longer by hanging my wet laundry to dry instead of using the dryer. It really does help with wear and tear, especially pilling of fabrics. So when I do shop again, buying used clothing will be greener than buying new organic or sustainable clothing. And yes, lots cheaper!

—Jan, 54, Johnson City, Tennessee

Chapter 8

Jagged Little Pills: Medication

Our unhealthy diet and constant chemical exposures play major roles in why we're all so sick and getting sicker. But another important factor is our drug-obsessed culture. For most people, it just seems easier and more convenient to pop a pill that soothes their symptoms instead of trying to figure out the root of their various health problems. The new over-the-counter weight loss drug Alli is a prime example of this. Countless studies have shown that the best way to lose weight is to eat a healthy, plant-based diet and exercise regularly. But many folks would rather pay good money to take a drug associated with a host of unpleasant side effects, from diarrhea to a potential increase in your risk for cancer! It just seems like the easy fix.

It's no surprise that bottles of Alli have sold like hotcakes—the pharmaceutical industry is very powerful and very skilled at convincing us that these easy fixes are the way to go. At least one hundred new prescription and over-the-counter drugs are introduced to our pharmacy shelves each year, reports the Natural Resources Defense Council's *OnEarth* magazine. More than 135 million of us use prescription drugs each month (adding up to over 4 billion prescriptions filled in 2004), a figure that represents a more than 100-percent increase since 2000, say researchers at the Teleosis Institute, a nonprofit organization based in

Berkeley, California, devoted to reducing the environmental impact of health care.

I'm not here to argue that we should give up all pharmaceuticals. In my work with the children who visit the Deirdre Imus Environmental Center for Pediatric Oncology at Hackensack University Medical Center and the Imus Ranch, I've seen drugs save and sustain hundreds of lives. But until we get to the bottom of the environmental issues that are making us so sick, these drugs are at best a Band-Aid solution to a much bigger problem. And at worst, pharmaceuticals can even contribute to the environment-wide toxicity that is making us sick in the first place, whether it's the chemicals they're concocted with, the ill effects they can have on us, or what happens to them after we're finished with them. To explain what I mean, I'm going to walk you through the life cycle of a typical drug.

Activist Spotlight

Earth Keepers and the Superior Watershed Partnership

On April 21, 2007, more than two thousand residents of Michigan's Upper Peninsula took the time to clean out their bathroom cabinets and drop off more than a ton of unwanted pills, powders, and liquid medicines. What inspired this earth -friendly spring cleaning? The largest drug take-back program ever organized in the United States, thanks to the devoted efforts of volunteers at 140 churches, synagogues, and other religious institutions. They're all part of Earth Keepers, a coalition of environmentalists from nine different faiths brought together by the Superior Watershed Partnership, a nonprofit organization in Marquette, Michigan, devoted to preserving the Great Lakes and the rivers and watersheds of the Upper Peninsula. "The EPA approached us and said that they thought a drug take-back program could be a really effective way of raising awareness and reducing the amount of medications that are currently polluting our waters," explains Natasha Koss, SWP's development coordinator, who oversaw the recruitment of volunteers at nineteen take-back sites. "We began to do our research and learned that the disposal of medication isn't just an environmental issue, it's also a public health concern and a law-enforcement issue." This is because tossing drugs in the trash increases the risk for a child or pet to be poisoned, as well as the risk for abuse—law enforcement officers at the take-back sites collected $500,000 worth of narcotics, while pharmacists handled prescription and over-the-counter medications. Earth Keepers arranged for the collected drugs to be incinerated at an environmentally friendly facility where emissions are cleaned to prevent air pollution. For more information on their efforts visit www .superiorwatersheds.org. For a toolkit to help you organize a drug take-back program in your own community, visit www .iisgcp.org/unwantedmeds.

Lifecycle Phase 1: Biopharming

When you swallow a pill, it probably doesn't occur to you to wonder where its ingredients—the powders, gels, chemicals, and fillers—came from. But if you heard your drugs were made from corn and potatoes, you might think that's a good thing—"natural" is better, right? Wrong. There's nothing natural about crops that have been genetically engineered to produce chemical reactions that Mother Nature never intended. It seems likely that the industrial farming of such crops will pose the same environmental risks as the industrial farming of food crops—a reduction in biodiversity, an increase in the use of pesticides, and so on. And we have no idea (because the biotech companies aren't required to tell us) what can happen to human health if these pharma crops accidentally enter our food supply. As Gregory Jaffe, director of the Center for Science in the Public Interest's Biotechnology Project explained in a June 2004 report called *Sowing Secrecy: The Biotech Industry, USDA, and America's Secret Pharm Belt*: "The USDA does not conduct an individual environmental risk assessment before it issues a permit [to biotech companies wishing to grow such crops], and none of an applicant's data on environmental risks is provided to the public . . . The FDA does not conduct a food-safety risk assessment prior to or after commercialization of a pharma crop and has no authority to prevent a crop that might endanger the food supply from being planted." But we do know that the risk for such contamination is real: In November 2002, the U.S. Department of Agriculture disclosed to the public that it was investigating ProdiGene, a biotechnology company that was producing a pig vaccine from corn, for possible violations of government-mandated permit conditions established to prevent their corn from escaping into the environment or contaminating the food supply at sites in Iowa and Nebraska.

The company denied doing anything wrong, but it agreed to pay a fine, and the USDA modified regulations so that all plants engineered to produce a pharmaceutical or industrial chemical would require a permit before they could be grown. But the entire process is still so shrouded in secrecy that there's really no way for you to know if the pills you're taking are coming from a pharma crop or a test tube. Their use runs the gamut from insulin produced by safflower plants, a hepatitis B vaccine produced from tobacco, a cholera vaccine from potatoes, and human serum albumin (used as blood volume replacement to treat patients suffering from shock and serious burns and during surgery) derived from corn, according to Jaffe's report.

My bottom line on pharma crops? Buyers beware. We desperately need more research and more regulation about how and if these genetically engineered plants should be used. In the meantime, continue to say no to GMOs whenever you do see them in food and other goods.

Lifecycle Phase 2: Drug Development

Whether a drug is synthetic or natural, the pharmaceutical industry wastes about 100 kilograms of raw materials for every 1 kilogram of active pharmaceutical ingredient produced, reports Niyati Desai, editorial director of *Symbiosis: The Journal of Ecologically Sustainable Medicine* published by the Teleosis Institute: (teleosis.org). This huge waste of natural resources is just the beginning of the pharmaceutical industry's negative environmental impacts. Consider these facts from Desai's 2007 report:

- Pharmaceutical manufacturers consume almost $1 billion in energy per year.

- In 2005, the average pharmaceutical company used more than 5 billion gallons of fresh water.

- The pharmaceutical giant GlaxoSmithKline alone disposed of 68 million kilograms of hazardous waste in 2005.

The good news: Several pharmaceutical companies have begun to green their production practices. Both Pfizer and Merck have been honored by the Environmental Protection Agency and other environmental organizations for their efforts to reduce waste and energy and water use. Some companies are recycling up to 90 percent of water used in production processes for landscaping purposes, notes Desai, as well as recycling solvents used during drug manufacturing and installing equipment to minimize the release of volatile organic compounds (VOCs) that are emitted during production. Although you don't always have a choice about who manufactures the drug you need, if your doctor does give you a few treatment options, all else being equal, I think it's important to support companies making an effort to reduce the eco footprint of their production processes.

Lifecycle Phase 3: Unexpected Impacts

From Vioxx and heart attacks, to the possible link between thimerosal vaccines and autism, I could give you countless examples of medications that were developed with the goal of improving human health but are, in fact, suspected of having caused great harm. Every year, more than 9.6 million adverse drug reactions occur in older Americans, say the researchers at www.worstpills.org. Whenever you're considering whether to take a new drug, I encourage you to do your homework first. To find out more about any particular drug, I recommend these excellent resources:

- **Worstpills.org.** This Web site is run by Public Citizen's Health Research Group, a nonprofit organization that accepts no advertising of any kind and no funding from government or corporations. It's directed by Sidney Wolfe, MD, an adjunct professor of internal medicine at the Case Western Reserve University School of Medicine. Dr. Wolfe and his team continually update this comprehensive site with the latest safety information on thousands of prescription drugs. A wealth of useful information is available for free, or for a fifteen-dollar annual subscription you can access their rigorous scientific analyses of specific drugs to understand why you should avoid them.

- **Prescription for Change.** This campaign, led by the renowned nonprofit Consumers Union (publisher of *Consumer Reports* and a major consumer-rights advocacy group), provides consumers with timely information about prescription drug issues and current efforts at the state and federal level to improve safety, effectiveness, and access to medicines (www.consumersunion.org/campaigns/prescription/about.html).

- Consumer Reports **Best Buy Drugs.** Prescription for Change's sister Web site provides free guidance on hundreds of prescription drugs. You can search by disease or brand name for up-to-date information on a drug's safety and efficacy, as well as access tons of money-saving tips (www.crbestbuydrgs.org).

Spotlight On: Birth Control

There are so many drugs with potential health risks and safety concerns that I could fill this entire book (and several more) discussing them. For information on drugs pertaining to children's health and fertility, I suggest you consult *Green This! Volume Two: Greening Baby;* the Web sites listed above will give you information about most other medications on the market. Here I've decided to highlight hormonal contraceptives because more than 10 million American women take birth control pills daily, making them one of the most-prescribed drugs in use today.

There's no question that the Pill revolutionized our society and gives women a phenomenal level of freedom and control over their lives. Unfortunately, we're still learning about the potential health ramifications of hormonal contraception, and the risks may be greater than we first thought. The main concern is that taking a hormonal contraceptive, whether it's a pill, patch, or ring, increases your body's exposure to synthetic estrogen.

"When we're left to our own devices, our bodies do a pretty good job of regulating the amount of estrogen in our system, as well as how our bodies respond to it. We have receptors designed to help ensure that we maintain the estrogen levels we need to keep our reproductive systems healthy and functioning, and if we get too much, our bodies turn some of those receptors off," explains Mady Hornig, MD, an associate professor of epidemiology at Columbia University's Mailman School of Public Health. "But there are so many environmental exposures to estrogen and chemicals that mimic or disrupt our natural estrogens that there is only so much adaptation that our systems can manage. And we know that a woman's lifetime risk for breast cancer is directly linked to her lifetime level of exposure to estrogen."

In addition to potentially increasing your risk for breast cancer, hormonal contraception is increasingly being linked to an elevated risk for clots in your larger blood vessels, particularly in smokers, notes Dr. Hornig. Of course there are many personal factors you will have to weigh when choosing the best birth control method for you. But whenever possible, Dr. Hornig advises women to consider nonhormonal forms of birth control, such as condoms, diaphragms, or the intrauterine device (IUD).

Another reason to rethink your use of hormonal contraceptives: They leave a heavy eco footprint. When you first slap an Ortho Evra birth control patch on your arm, it contains 6 milligrams of the synthetic hormone norelgestromin and 0.60 milligrams of ethinyl estradiol, a synthetic estrogen. Your body, to prevent pregnancy, absorbs some of those hormones. But when you toss the patch in the trash or flush it down the toilet at the end of the week, a whopping 76 to 82 percent of the original hormone content is still there, according to a 2004 report by the Canadian nonprofit group Women and Health Protection. Those remaining hormones are just waiting to be released into our ecosystem as soon as that patch makes its way to your local municipal landfill or sewage system, and studies have shown that these hormones can feminize male fish.

NuvaRing, a contraceptive rubber ring worn inside a woman's vagina, then discarded at the end of each menstrual cycle, may be even worse. WHP reports that a discarded ring still contains a third more synthetic estrogen than a month's worth of discarded patches and up to six times as much hormone as a month's supply of birth control pills. These hormonal methods are popular because they are so much more convenient than remembering to take a pill each day—but it's just too soon to tell what these super-sized doses of synthetic hormones are really doing to your body, or to the environment once they make their way out.

Lifecycle Phase 4: Drug Disposal

I know what you're thinking: The few milligrams of hormones that remain when you toss your birth control patch in the trash each week can hardly be enough to really turn male fish female or have any significant environmental impact. It's just a little tiny dose of estrogen, right?

Well, consider this: Millions of other women are also tossing their birth control patches in the trash every week, week after week, and year after year. And that's in addition to the numerous other kinds of medication that enter the waste stream via our trash cans, toilets, and drains. Patch by patch and pill by pill, our drug-obsessed culture is adding up to what the EPA describes as one of the most significant emerging environmental threats of the twenty-first century. Residues from medication (and other personal-care products such as our shampoos, sunscreens and fragrances; refer back to chapter 5 for more details) now pollute almost every source of water around the globe.

The EPA calculates that drug residues have probably been polluting our waters as long as we've been using (and excreting or discarding) them. But it wasn't until the last decade that technology advanced to the point where scientists could detect their presence, as it's usually at very low levels (described as parts per billion or even parts per trillion). As a result, it's still too soon to say definitively what effect chronic exposure to low levels of drugs is having on our environment or on our health. But scientists say there are good reasons to be concerned. For one thing, drugs are designed to work at the lowest dose possible—so even very small levels of exposure may well effect us if they are consistent, and the possibility of unintended side effects at subtherapeutic doses cannot be discounted. Although many pharmaceutical ingredients degrade quickly in the environment, our high rates of drug use ensure that we are constantly replenishing the supply. Christian Daughton, PhD, chief of the Environmental Chemistry Branch of the EPA in Las Vegas, Nevada, notes that while it's straightforward enough to study the effects of a single drug in a lab setting, it's currently not possible to study how multiple drugs interact with one another at extremely low concentrations with other pollutants in our environment—but that's exactly the kind of chemical cocktail with which we're spiking our water.

Environmental Toll

What kind of negative effects do we know about? Fish, frogs, and other aquatic species have become our canaries in this new coal mine, and the preliminary data are alarming:

- Antidepressants known as selective serotonin reuptake inhibitors (SSRIs) have the potential to adversely impact how shellfish spawn, even at low parts-per-billion concentrations, notes Daughton.

- Calcium-channel blockers (used to relieve chest pain and hypertension) can dramatically inhibit the sperm activity of some aquatic organisms, says the EPA.

- David Norris, an environmental endocrinologist at the University of Colorado at Boulder, found that female white suckers, a kind of bottom-feeding fish, outnumber males by more than five to one in Boulder Creek, and that 50 percent of males have some female sex tissue. Similar intersex changes have been found in flathead chubs and smallmouth bass. The cause, Norris suspects, is exposure to estrogen, which isn't designed to break down easily, has effects at low dosages with chronic use, and only partially dissolves in water.

- Baylor University researchers found tiny amounts of Prozac in liver and brain tissue of channel catfish and black crappie captured in a creek near Dallas, reports *OnEarth* magazine. A University of Georgia scientist found that tadpoles exposed to Prozac morphed into undersize frogs, which are vulnerable to predation and environmental stress.

- More than two hundred species—aquatic and terrestrial— are known or suspected to have experienced adverse reactions to endocrine disruptors like estrogen and its synthetic mimics, according to a report by the Scientific Committee on Problems of the Environment, a worldwide network of scientists and scientific institutions, and the International Union of Pure and Applied Chemistry.

Human Toll

As we learn more about what these drug residues are doing to our aquatic life, researchers are beginning to connect the dots to potential human health impacts as well. For instance, a survey of cancer rates in Hardy County, Virginia, where some residents drink from the same water inhabited by intersex fish, found rates of cancer of the liver, gallbladder, ovaries, and uterus were all higher than the state average, reports the *Washington Post*. Says *OnEarth* magazine: "In the United Kingdom, hormones in the environment have been linked with lowered sperm counts and gynecomastia—the development of breasts in men." And don't forget about our toxic cocktail: A mix of thirteen medications commonly found in drinking water was shown to inhibit cell growth in human embryonic cells even at low concentrations, according to a landmark 2006 study published in the *Environmental Science and Technology*.

The potential for damage to an embryo and thus a growing fetus is what concerns and angers me most, especially when I consider the precautions that so many pregnant women take to minimize chemical exposures that might harm their developing child. Toxicologists worry about pregnant mothers having unintended exposure to drugs they are told to avoid during pregnancy, says Dr. Daughton.

Green Your Drug Disposal

Here's how to use and dispose of your drugs more safely:

1. Minimize your need for pharmaceuticals by greening your diet and reducing your chemical exposures whenever possible. Exercise regularly, use vitamins and herbal supplements (more on these in chapter 9) to promote good health, and don't smoke.

2. Purchase drugs in small amounts. Ask for the smallest prescription size unless you're treating a chronic condition. With over-the-counter drugs, only buy as much cold medicine as you need to treat your current cold, for instance. The megasize bottle will just go to waste if you can't use it all before it expires.

3. Ask your doctor and pharmacist about the environmental impacts of your medication and whether a more sustainable alternative exists. Look for recycled packaging when choosing over-the-counter brands. You can get more information on this at the Teleosis Insititute (teleosis.org).

4. Don't flush unused medications down the toilet, unless the label specifically instructs you to do so or unless they are on the following list of drugs that the Food and Drug Administration says should be flushed to minimize the risk of abuse:

-   Actiq (fentanyl citrate)
-   Daytrana transdermal patch (methylphenidate)
-   Duragesic transdermal system (fentanyl)
-   OxyContin tablets (oxycodone)
-   Avinza capsules (morphine sulfate)
-   Baraclude tablets (entecavir)
-   Reyataz capsules (atazanavir sulfate)
-   Tequin tablets (gatifloxacin)
-   Zerit for oral solution (stavudine)
-   Meperidine HCl tablets

- Percocet (oxycodone and Acetaminophen)

- Xyrem (sodium oxybate)

- Fentora (fentanyl buccal tablet)

5. Look for a take-back program instead of disposing of drugs yourself. Your doctor's office, pharmacy, or community center may sponsor a program that discards drugs in an environmentally friendly manner or redistributes unused medications to nonprofit organizations in nonindustrial countries that need basic medication, say the experts at the Teleosis Institute.

6. If you do toss medications in the trash, crush or dissolve the drugs in water and mix with kitty litter, sawdust, coffee grounds, or any other material that absorbs the drug and makes it less appealing for pets or children to eat, then place in a sealed plastic bag.

Green (and Clean!) Your Water

Each July, local water departments send every homeowner a consumer confidence report (if you rent, check with your landlord). This pamphlet will tell you how your water rates in terms of "regulated substances," the chemicals that the EPA monitors because they pose health risks. Any chemical that exceeds the EPA safety limit will be flagged as a violation and is something you'll want to filter out. The CCR also tells you the level of "turbidity," or cloudiness in your water, which can indicate the presence of disease-causing microorganisms if the level is too high. If you have questions about your water quality, call your local water supplier or the EPA's Safe Drinking Water Hotline

(800.426.4791). I subscribe wholeheartedly to the precautionary principle, so I think that installing a water filter in your house is a great way to reduce the number of toxins that you and your family encounter every day.

Most water suppliers do not yet test for drug residues, because they lack the expensive technology required to monitor chemicals at such low levels. But the EPA's Dr. Daughton notes, "One of the most effective approaches for consumer filtration of water is a technology called 'reverse osmosis' (RO). A variety of commercial RO units are available, which are highly effective at removing the vast majority of all water constituents." So while there's no way to know for sure that you are removing drug residues from your water, an RO filter will take care of lead, chlorine, chloroform, sediment, mercury, dissolved solids (minerals like sodium and calcium), arsenic, nitrates, fluoride, and bad tastes.

RO filters work by using pressure to pump water through a membrane that separates out contaminants. Keep in mind that the system is only effective as long as it's properly maintained—you'll need to change the filter cartridges periodically and replace the membrane itself according to the manufacturer's guidelines. "When any point-of-use water treatment device used by consumer is not properly maintained, it has the potential to actually degrade the quality of the water, because of microbial growth inside the device and because of 'breakthrough' of high concentrations of contaminants once a cartridge has been saturated," warns Dr. Daughton. RO systems are also bulky (most are installed under your kitchen sink) and expensive ($200 to $300 for the initial device, plus $50 to $75 per year in maintenance costs).

A more convenient and less expensive filtration option is to purchase a pitcher, carafe, or water cooler that uses an activated carbon filter (AC). When you fill the pitcher with tap water, the carbon filter acts like a magnet, drawing impurities to its surface while the water passes through. Most pitcher-style AC filters will remove lead, chlorine, chloroform, sediment, mercury, benzene, and bad tastes and odors and are relatively inexpensive ($25 to $35, though you will need to replace the filter frequently). You can also find AC filters that attach to your sink's faucet and will remove some pesticides in addition to the above list; more expensive under-sink models can also handle VOCs, if your consumer confidence report says those are a problem in your area. But in general, AC filters will be slightly less efficient than RO models, can slow down your water pressure if you're using a faucet or under-sink model, and require vigilance to replace filters frequently.

Whatever kind of filter you choose, look for a model that has been certified by NSF International (formerly the National Sanitation Foundation, nsf.org), a nonprofit organization that sets industry standards for regulating the effectiveness of filters. This is your only guarantee that a filter will do what it promises. For a list of trustworthy water filters, see my Eco Shopping List on page 205.

Lifecycle Phase 5: Antibiotic Resistance

No discussion of the environmental impact of the pharmaceutical industry would be complete without a look at the rapidly developing problem of antibiotic resistance. The more we use antibiotics, the more we contribute to the rise of antibiotic-resistant bacteria. Penicillin, ciprofloxacin, and other antibiotics are designed to kill the bacteria that make us sick, but whenever we use them, a tiny fraction of the bacteria may have the ability to survive. "When the antibiotic kills off their competitors, only the resistant bacteria multiply. And they can pass their resistance on to their offspring and to other types of bacteria," report researchers at Center for Science in the Public Interest.

I think consumers often view antibiotic resistance as some kind of futuristic sci-fi problem, but we're already starting to feel its effects. Diseases such as tuberculosis, gonorrhea, malaria, and childhood ear infections are now more difficult to treat than they were just a few decades ago, reports the National Institute of Allergy and Infectious Diseases (NIAID). The CSPI notes that one in six *Campylobacter* infections (the type of bacteria responsible for most cases of food poisoning) are now resistant to fluoroquinolone antibiotics like Cipro, which are used in both humans and poultry. And one in five urinary tract infections are now resistant to Bactrim, the antibiotic usually used to treat them. This means doctors must use Cipro or another equally at-risk drug on these common infections. In our hospitals, about 90,000 patients die each year as a result of a bacterial infection they acquire during their stay, up from 13,300 patient deaths in 1992. NIAID attributes the increase to the fact that more than 70 percent of the bacteria that cause hospital-acquired infections are now resistant to at least one of the antibiotics most commonly used to treat them. And at some point, we may simply run out of antibiotics that work.

I'm also concerned about a less-publicized side effect of antibiotics: their role in increasing our risk for breast cancer. A February 2004 study by Seattle-based oncologists published in the *Journal of the American Medical Association (JAMA)* studied the use of antibiotics among 10,219 women, 2,266 of whom had developed breast cancer. They found that risk of breast cancer doubled in those who had used antibiotics for more than five hundred cumulative days. The risk was the same whether a respiratory tract or skin infection was being treated. A similar epidemiological study, published in 2000, looked at breast-cancer patients in Finland. In a study population of ten thousand women, investigators found that women younger than fifty who reported having taken antibiotics for urinary-tract infections had elevated rates of breast cancer compared with women who didn't use antibiotics. While some very strong antibiotics—chloramphenicol or fluorquinolone for example—are proven carcinogens, the Seattle researchers also looked at such commonly prescribed antibiotics as tetracycline, erythromycin, penicillin VK, and cephalexin, which are not thought to be carcinogenic. What the studies don't reveal is if the increased cancer rates are due to a function of the drugs (antibiotics may interfere with our bodies' absorption of cancer-fighting nutrients, for instance), the age of the women when they took the drugs, or some common denominator among the underlying infections.

Whatever the end result, there are plenty of excellent reasons for us to be more cautious about our use of antibiotics, starting now. Here's what you can do:

1. Avoid unnecessary antibiotics. "People who have taken antibiotics recently are more susceptible to infections with bacteria that are resistant and may pass them on to family members and friends," say the experts at CSPI. And remember that many common illnesses are caused by viruses, not bacteria, and will not respond to antibiotics, including:

    •   Most sore throats (though strep throat is caused by bacteria, so ask your doctor for a throat culture to determine what's causing your symptoms before you start medication)

    •   Colds

    •   Flu

    •   Coughs

    •   Bronchitis (but if your symptoms last more than two weeks, or if you have a lung condition, your symptoms may be caused by bacteria)

    •   Many ear infections

- Sinus infections (as long as they do not last longer than two weeks)

2. Take antibiotics as directed. If you stop taking the antibiotic early because you're feeling better, the bacteria that are still alive can restart an infection.
3. Do not save antibiotics for later or share them with others. Using only part of a prescription could allow the bacteria that survive the treatment to reinfect you.
4. Choose organic if you eat meat, to reduce your intake of antibiotics and hormones and to support the green livestock and poultry industries that do not contribute to antibiotic resistance.
5. Don't buy antibacterial soaps. They're no more effective at getting rid of germs than plain soap. Instead, try a brand with essential oils, which are naturally antimicrobial, such as my Imus Greening the Cleaning hand and dish soaps.

Eco Shopping List

Here are some brands of water filters that have received the NSF seal. For more, visit www.nsf.org/Certified/DWTU/.

Reverse Osmosis Filters

- Kenmore 38575 Ultra Filter 450 Reverse Osmosis Drinking Water System, sears.com
- GE SmartWater GXRM10G, geappliances.com/smart water

Activated Carbon Filters

- Pūr Ultimate Slim Design Pitcher CR-800. purwater filter.com.

- Brita Faucet Filtration System OPFF-100, Brita.com.

- Brita Aquaview Faucet Filtration System, Brita.com.

- Pūr Ultimate Horizontal Faucet Mount FM-4900L purwaterfilter.com

---

A Greener You

Here's how readers like you are rethinking our drug-obsessed culture:

The other day I was trying to buy some liquid hand soap at the drugstore, and I literally could not find a single brand that wasn't 'antibacterial'! I like to take Dr. Bronner's liquid castile soap on trips because it's natural, biodegradable, and you can use it for so many things when you're traveling (shampoo, body wash, cleaning clothes, cleaning dishes and equipment when you're camping, etc.).

—Jen, 31, Brooklyn, New York

I am very concerned about the questionable ethics of many of the leading pharmaceutical companies. I am concerned that America is obsessed with quick fixes for everything. It seems like more than 50 percent of the advertising on television and in print is for prescription drugs! So I avoid OTC and prescription drugs. I try to let my illnesses run their course, or use herbal or nonchemical remedies.

—Priya, 39, Dublin, Ohio

I was diagnosed with Crohn's disease in 2000 and had been very sick off and on leading up to that point. Although I have always been one of those people who won't even take a Tylenol unless I really can't function, I never questioned my doctors much about the medications they wanted me to try. Since my diagnosis, however, I've made a complete turnaround in both my health and my attitude toward questioning my doctors. I am very careful about any kind of medication and always try an alternative, less invasive, path first. I strongly believe that no medication is without some kind of side effect. I rely a lot on an extensive supply of essential oils to help with everything from bug bites to headaches.

—Anjali, 38, Ardmore, Pennsylvania

Chapter 9

A New Kind of Medicine:
Alternative Remedies

With pharmaceutical drugs polluting our waters, and in some cases our bodies, trading in chemical-based medications for the natural world of alternative medicine might seem like a no-brainer. A big part of living a greener life is taking a more holistic approach to your health care, seeking out doctors and treatments that aren't just taking a Band-Aid, drug-based approach but are really going to heal your body. So let's take a closer look at alternative medicine and how it can benefit your health. (Remember that I'm not a doctor; always consult your own doctor or homeopath before trying any new treatment.)

Vitamins and Supplements

I am a fan of vitamins and herbal medicine and use supplements myself daily. But like all the other industries we've visited in this book, the $20 billion "nutraceuticals" industry is not always as consumer or environmentally friendly as we might like. As Marion Nestle, PhD, writes in her book *What to Eat*: "Supplement trade associations and companies work hard to convince you that your diet is deficient in nutrients, that this deficiency threatens your health, and that supplements are the solution to whatever ails you." So before you go wild in the aisles of your local Vitamin Shoppe or GNC, read this chapter.

Why Take Supplements?

If you eat a nutritious, plant-based diet and are generally healthy, you probably don't need to spend your money on a ton of pills and potions. But even if you eat the healthiest diet in the world, it's a sad fact of life on our now-toxic planet that the plant foods we're eating today aren't as nutrient rich as they used to be. Once again, it all comes down to our soil. As I discussed in chapter 2, corporate farming and other industries have depleted the nutritional content of our soil and this is directly impacting the quality of the food we grow. Improved nutrition, fortification of refined grains, and other public health initiatives have improved the situation somewhat, but not enough to keep pace with the environmental devastation that has continued unchecked. "Unfortunately, we all have a big job ahead to restore our soil quality— even on organic farms—and bring back the nutrients that have been farmed out of our food," writes Brian Clement, PhD, co-director of the Hippocrates Health Institute in West Palm Beach, Florida, in his book *The Vitamin Myth Exposed.* "It is urgent that we reintroduce proper organic farming as the primary method, as well as the rotation of crops to improve the quality of our soils, among other benefits. It has taken many decades to ruin our soils and it will take time to revive them and bring them back to health again . . . In the meantime, the way to guarantee adequate nutrition is by supplementing our foods with naturally-occurring, non-synthetic vitamin and nutrients from organic farms that focus on soil conservation."

Another great argument for dietary supplements: Nobody's perfect! I put a great deal of time and effort into making sure I eat an organic, plant-based diet, but even I have days or weeks where my schedule gets crazy. And alternative wellness guru Andrew Weil, MD, director of the Program in Integrative Medicine at the University of Arizona, does too: "Taking supplements does not excuse you from eating a healthy diet," he writes in his book *Healthy Aging: A Lifelong Guide to Your Well-Being.* "[But] I take a good daily multivitamin-multimineral supplement, one that I formulated myself, as insurance against gaps in my diet—for example, to cover those days when I am on the road and simply can't get the fruits and vegetables I'd like."

And when we do occasionally fall ill, nutritional supplements can often work wonders that whole foods aren't capable of, but without the same toxicity risks of most drugs. "Supplements can provide optimum dosages of natural therapeutic agents that may help prevent and treat age-related diseases," says Dr. Weil. "Many studies suggest that doses in the range of 200 to 400 IU of alpha-tocopherol [vitamin E] offer the best antioxidant protection against common age-related diseases. Nuts are good for you, but you would have to eat far too many of them to get that amount of vitamin E."

But before we talk about which supplements you should consider taking, there are a few issues you need to understand about the environmental health of the supplements industry today.

Eco Issue 1: Contamination

When you swallow a supplement tablet, it's reasonable to expect that the substances you just ingested are the same ones listed on the side of the bottle. But loopholes in the FDA's regulation of the dietary supplements industry mean that's not always the case. Tod Cooperman, MD, founded ConsumerLab.com in 1999 to fill in the gap, and to date his team has conducted tests on more than two thousand products. Check out their shocking discoveries:

- In a 2007 analysis of glucosamine and chondroitin supplements (used to treat osteoarthritis and joint pain), the majority of the products tested didn't contain as much chondroitin as advertised on the label. "The material suppliers were substituting cheaper compounds that look like chondroitin on some lab tests but aren't the real thing," Dr. Cooperman explains. "The brands selling these products either don't know what's going on [because their suppliers are responsible] or they don't want to know."

- In a review of St. John's wort products (an herb used to treat mild depression), many brands even some that were certified organic were found to have heavy metal contamination. "The organic seal may explain how an herb is grown, but we have found it does not assure purity," says Dr. Cooperman.

- On average, one in four of the supplements Consumer lab.com tests has a quality problem (contamination, too much of an ingredient, too little of an ingredient, or spoilage).

- Consumerlab.com isn't the only research group with these kinds of findings. Perchlorate (a chemical used in rocket fuel) was found in twenty of thirty-one vitamins tested by researchers at the Water Quality Research and Development Department of Southern Nevada in 2001.

What's going on? "Raw materials for supplements come from all over the world, including the USA, China, and India," explains Dr. Cooperman. "Contamination can happen in the ground where minerals are extracted or the soil where the herbs are grown. Certain plants accumulate heavy metals. Purity also depends on how the supplier processes the raw materials. The bottom line is that it's rare that we test a product line and find all of them to be fine."

Until the FDA tightens regulations (more on this starting on page 217), there's no way for you to know if a vitamin or supplement you're using is contaminated. "You could take a product for years and years and have no idea that it's contaminated. But some contaminants get stored in your body, such as lead which builds up in your bones," says Dr. Cooperman. "But most doctors wouldn't think to consider, say, your multivitamin as a source of exposure to lead."

Choose Safer Supplements

You can minimize your chances of buying a contaminated product with these tips.

- Buy organic, food-grade supplements. These are the least likely to have contamination issues.

- Avoid herbs grown in China. "They're more likely to be contaminated with pesticides, insecticides, and other substances," says Dr. Weil.

- Choose calcium citrate over calcium from oyster shells, which, according to Dr. Weil, may contain small amounts of lead.

- Do not exceed the recommended dosage. "Make sure you're taking the appropriate dose of a supplement for your condition," advises Dr. Cooperman. "The risks for side effects and even toxicity may increase with higher doses."

- Choose herbal extracts over whole herbs. "You'd think the whole herb is better, but, the extract may actually be cleaner because the extraction process removes many contaminants," says Dr. Cooperman.

- Look for products that bear the seal of the United States Pharmacopeia (USP), a public health organization. This ensures that the supplement has undergone rigorous independent testing and verification to vouch for the ingredients' integrity, purity, and potency. But keep in mind that the seal is only about quality control—it won't ensure that the product actually works the way it promises.

Eco Issue 2: The Great Synthetics Debate

As we've seen time and again in food and beauty products, "natural" can be a vague and relative term. The same goes for the supplements industry. Some products describe themselves as natural because they use yeast or algae as a base, to which synthetic vitamins and nutrients are added, while others mix synthetic dyes and fillers with plant extracts. As much as 90 percent of the average multivitamin tablet is pure filler, reports the Organic Consumers Association (OCA). "The OCA does not claim that synthetic vitamins are all totally useless," says the organization's director, Ronnie Cummins. "Some of these synthetics have their place in emergency health situations. But many are also unhealthy, and naturally occurring vitamins and minerals found in organic foods and 100-percent plant or food-based supplements are much better. Labeling synthetic ingredients as 'natural' is consumer fraud." I couldn't agree more. Consumers have a right to know what they're buying, and labeling a synthetic product as "natural" is yet another example of the greenwashing that wastes our time and money.

But beyond the importance of truth in advertising, how big a deal are synthetic supplements? It depends on the product. "Sometimes it doesn't matter," says Dr. Cooperman. "Vitamin C is the same compound, whether it's from synthetic ascorbic acid or rose hips." And "natural" doesn't always mean better. As we've already seen, natural herbs and minerals are just as prone to contamination as synthetics, if they are grown in unhealthy soil. It's also a common misconception that natural products are somehow less potent than synthetics. In fact, many pharmaceuticals are derived from plants that can have profound effects on our bodies, when used in concentrated doses—or incorrectly. Some manufacturers "sell traditional herbal medicines for non-traditional purposes," said Bruce Silverglade, legal affairs director for the CSPI. "A herb that may have produced minimal side effects when used for a traditional purpose may cause severe adverse reactions when used for a different purpose." Don't assume a product is safe just because the manufacturer tells you "it has been used in China for hundreds of years!"

Furthermore, not all natural ingredients are ones you would want to ingest. In 2001, the Associated Press reported that Scott Norton, MD, a Maryland physician, discovered the presence of brains, testicles, tracheas, and glands from cows and other animals in several dietary supplements. While FDA officials contended that "the issue isn't a huge concern" because the majority of supplements are made from plants, not animals, and most bovine-containing supplements are made from "safe" U.S. cattle, these are not products that I would take.

But there's no question that many synthetic supplements can be hazardous to your health. Beware of these potential risks:

- **Mega-Dosing.** Synthetic supplements tend to contain enormous doses of vitamins and minerals—often more than your body can handle. This isn't too much of a concern with water-soluble vitamins (vitamin C and eight B vitamins), which flush out of your system quite easily. But some vitamins, including A, D, E, and K, are fat soluble. This means they tend to build up in your body's fat tissues and liver. If you're regularly ingesting more than the recommended daily allowance (RDA) of these vitamins, you could end up overdosing and making yourself quite sick.

"When [the body] is saturated with large amounts of synthetic vitamins . . . it will then work to eliminate them through the kidneys, skin, and other elimination organs," writes Dr. Clement. The best-case scenario is that your body will succeed in eliminating the vitamins—but before they can offer you any health benefits. In the worst case, your system can't eliminate the megadoses quickly enough and you suffer from acute toxicity. "One easy way to tell [if the supplement is synthetic] is to look at the RDA," advises the OCA. "If the potency is higher than anything you would find in nature (say, 1,000 % RDA of vitamin C per serving), then the product contains synthetically produced ingredients, no matter what the producer of the product might claim."

- **Nanoparticles.** Just as beauty companies are adding these tiny but potent forms of ingredients to cosmetics and sunscreens, supplement makers have found they can boost sales by shrinking their ingredients down to a smaller size, reports the OCA. See chapters 5 and 6 for a detailed discussion of the health risks of nanoparticles—needless to say, if they're dangerous when applied to your skin, they may be even worse when you swallow them whole.

- **Petrochemicals.** Many synthetic supplements, particularly B vitamins, are made from ingredients derived from petroleum, reports the OCA. "Crystalline yellow coal tar derived from fossil fuel sources," the same carcinogen found in hair dyes and dandruff shampoos, is another popular base material, says Dr. Clement. See chapters 5 and 6 for more details on why you should avoid these.

- **Allergens.** Many people are allergic to coal tar and other chemicals used as base ingredients for synthetic vitamins, reports the OCA. Ingredients to avoid if you're allergy prone: nicotine, alloxal, magnesium stearate, stearic acid, silicon dioxide ("common sand used as an expensive filler to make the bottle weigh more with the hope that the uneducated consumer will equate weight with higher quality," says OCA), natural flavors (which could mean MSG), methylcellulose, carnauba wax, and titanium dioxide.

- **Synthetic Vitamin E.** While Dr. Weil notes that "synthetics tend to work just as well" for most supplements, "the exception is vitamin E. Nature produces vitamin E as a complex of eight molecules, and most supplements only give you one, in a synthetic form, only half of which is useful to the body."

Choose Safer Supplements

Although scientists debate the extent to which synthetic supplements are dangerous, I like to play it safe. Whenever you have the choice, choose 100-percent organic, plant-based, food-grade products over synthetic. "Look for the phrase 'naturally occurring,'" advises Dr. Clement, noting that the ingredient list should also name the food source of each nutrient. Your best bet is to choose supplements that have been certified by the Naturally Occurring Standards Group, an independent certification organization run by Dr. Clement's Hippocrates Health Institute and the OCA.

Eco Issue 3: The FDA

Why is it so easy for supplement manufacturers to get away with mislabeled, unnatural, and even toxic products? Once again, we must take a hard look at the relationship between industry and our government's regulatory body, the Food and Drug Administration. When it comes to marketing a vitamin, mineral, or herbal supplement, pretty much anything goes: "While visiting a game park in South Africa in 2005, I learned that elephant dung is used locally as a remedy for migraine headaches. All I would have to do to market a supplement made from this substance . . . would be to inform the FDA that I am selling this 'new dietary ingredient' and explain why it might reasonably be expected to be safe," writes Dr. Marion Nestle. "As long as not too many people die from eating this product, no federal agency is going to pay much attention."

The regulation is particularly loose regarding the risk for contamination. "It's really up to the manufacturer to determine the level of quality in their products and the type of testing they conduct," says Dr. Cooperman. "The FDA is not checking products for lead and other contaminants on any regular basis." If the FDA does learn of a contamination issue (often thanks to ConsumerLab.com testing), they do have the power to remove dangerous products from store shelves. But they must first prove that the products pose "a significant or unreasonable risk," which usually means waiting for people to get sick.

The FDA also fails to monitor closely the claims manufacturers can make about their products because it does not require premarket testing for dietary supplements the way it does for pharmaceutical drugs— it simply forbids manufacturers from making a definitive claim about a product's ability to prevent, cure, or treat a disease. As a result, a lot of ill-supported claims slip through the cracks. Silverglade's testimony pointed to garlic, an herb "widely promoted for maintaining heart health and/or healthy cholesterol levels. Typical claims include statements such as 'regular consumption of garlic may help promote healthy heart function and regulate cholesterol levels.'" But an evidence review by the Agency for Healthcare Research and Quality found that garlic's benefits last no longer than six months, which garlic supplement manufacturers aren't required to reveal—even though, Silverglade explained, "it is *prolonged* elevation of blood cholesterol levels that raises the risk of cardiovascular disease. Thus, a product that does not work beyond six months is virtually useless." Unless you're willing to pay to stay on it for the rest of your life.

Of course the upshot of such poor safety guarantees and suspect health claims is that consumers stop buying, which is a shame because many supplements provide real health benefits. Public health advocates are working to prevent this by pushing the FDA to clean up its act. "I would like to see the FDA create a new division of natural therapeutic agents to regulate herbs, vitamins, minerals, and other products to ensure that products on the market are safe, contain what they claim to contain, and do what they claim to do," says Dr. Weil.

We have made some progress. In 2006, Congress approved the Dietary Supplement and Nonprescription Drug Consumer Protection

Act, requiring manufacturers to list an address or telephone number on product labels that consumers can use to report serious adverse reactions—and making it mandatory for manufacturers to then disclose such reports to the FDA. "Under the previous voluntary system, the FDA received less than 1 percent of all reports of adverse reactions to dietary supplements," says Silverglade.

The FDA also announced that they would begin requiring manufacturers to follow good manufacturing practices (GMPs), which include provisions for manufacturing operations, quality control procedures, testing of raw materials and final products, and the design and construction of manufacturing plants to facilitate maintenance. "The rule will give consumers greater confidence that the dietary supplement they use has been manufactured to ensure its identity, purity, strength, and composition," announced the FDA in June 2007.

But we still have a long way to go. "These regulations will not ensure that supplements are safe and effective," says CSPI staff attorney Ilene Heller. "Nor will the GMPs address whether the products carry adequate directions for use and appropriate warnings." And though the act of Congress requires manufacturers to report adverse reactions, the FDA is only required to inspect high-risk companies. "Given the FDA's limited resources, that may be as infrequently as once every five years," notes Heller.

Supplement Shopping List

Between dubious research, lack of regulation, misleading labels, and potential risk for contamination, you might decide you're better off without any supplements in your diet, thanks all the same. But I do think, and many leading health experts agree, that there is an important place for supplements in a healthy lifestyle, as a kind of health insurance policy and to treat certain nutrient deficiencies and health problems. The key is to do your research before you buy. Be wary of any supplement that becomes very popular very quickly. "That's going to be a hearsay situation," warns Dr. Cooperman. Look for the USP certification seal, avoid synthetic ingredients and megadoses, and research any new supplement to see if it really can do what it promises. Some excellent sources for more information:

- **ConsumerLab.com.** Because Cooperman's organization does not accept advertising, it costs thirty dollars per year to subscribe, but I think it's well worth the investment to be able to access their wealth of reports and information.

- **PDR for Nutritional Supplements, Sheldon S. Hendler and David Rorvik.** This research-based review of supplements "does the best they can with the limited science available," says Dr. Nestle.

- **National Institutes of Health's Office of Dietary Supplements (http:dietary-supplements.info.nih. gov).** Here you can obtain fact sheets on vitamins, minerals, and herbal supplements, as well as check for updates on research and get tips on avoiding supplement scams.

- **HerbalGram (herbalgram.org).** The journal of the American Botanical Council publishes the latest scientific studies on the effectiveness of plant-based medicine.

- **Consumer Reports (consumerreports.org).** The magazine of the nonprofit Consumers Union regularly assesses the effectiveness and safety of popular supplements.

- **Nutrition Action Health Letter (cspinet.org).** The nutritionists who publish CSPI's newsletter perform rigorous analyses of groups of supplements and frequently list their top picks and products to avoid.

Now here are the supplements I think are worth considering. You'll want to shop around to find brands that fit your needs and budget, but four that I think are quite trustworthy are Bluebonnet (bluebonnetnutrition.com), New Chapter (new-chapter.com), Spectrum (spectrumorganics.com), and Weil (drweil.com). I'll also buy empty vegetarian gel capsules from the health food store and fill them with essential oils like lemon, clove, and thyme—great for travel. As always, consult your personal health care practitioner before adopting these or any other suggestions involving supplements.

Multivitamin/Multimineral

"Everyone should take one of these," says Dr. Weil. "It covers gaps in your diet and is especially important if you're not eating enough fruits and vegetables." You can take yours any time of day, but be sure to take it on a full stomach, to avoid indigestion and make sure the fat-soluble vitamins can be properly absorbed. There are a million multis on the market, so here's Dr. Weil's checklist of what makes a good one:

- No: Synthetic, preformed vitamin A (retinol)
- Yes: A mixture of carotenoids (not just beta-carotene, which can be dangerous on its own), which includes lutein, lycopene, and other antioxidant pigments

- Yes: Vitamin E as mixed, natural tocopherol (not synthetic dl-alpha-tocopherol), with mixed tocotrienols, the other components in the natural vitamin E complex

- Yes: 50 milligrams each of most B vitamins; at least 400 micrograms of folic acid; at least 50 micrograms of vitamin B_{12}

- No: More than 200 milligrams of vitamin C (that's all your body can use in a day)

- Yes: 400 to 1,000 IU of vitamin D

- No: Iron, unless you are a menstruating woman, pregnant, or have documented iron-deficiency anemia

- No: More than 200 micrograms of selenium

- Yes: Calcium, preferably calcium citrate

The rest of these are optional, but worth knowing about, as you might find they'll play an important role in maintaining your health.

Alpha-Lipoic Acid (With or Without Acetyl-L-Carnitine)

"This antioxidant is interesting to me because it decreases insulin resistance while augmenting the body's antioxidant defenses," says Dr. Weil. "If you have any degree of metabolic syndrome (low HDL cholesterol, high serum triglycerides, a tendency to gain weight in the abdomen, a tendency toward high blood pressure) or have a personal or family history of obesity or type 2 diabetes, it might be worth taking ALA. Start with 100 milligrams a day; you can take up to 400 milligrams a day."

Vitamin B_{12}

If you're vegan, you may want to supplement additional B_{12} in your diet because it's hard to get enough from plant foods grown in depleted soils. (For more details, refer to chapter 3.) I take 5,000 micrograms of Bluebonnet methylcobalamin vitamin B_{12} daily. It's free of milk, eggs, fish, crustacean shellfish, nuts, peanuts, wheat, yeast, barley, rice, sodium, and soybeans.

CoQ10 (Coenzyme Q or Ubiquinone)

This antioxidant increases oxygen use at the cellular level, improving the function of heart muscle cells and boosting capacity for aerobic exercise, says Dr. Weil. "It is much researched and widely used. I take it myself, and frequently recommend it to patients, including those with cancer, diabetes, and gum disease." He recommends 60 milligrams a day in a soft-gel formula, which is easier for your body to absorb, especially if you're on statin drugs, which inhibit your body's natural production.

Fish Oil

"If you're not eating oily fish at least twice a week, take supplemental fish oil in capsule or liquid form," says Dr. Weil, who recommends 1 to 2 grams daily to help protect your cardiovascular and neurological health. Look for molecularly distilled products certified to be free of heavy metals and other contaminants.

Folic Acid (For Women)

If you're thinking about becoming pregnant, you should take an additional 400 micrograms of folic acid daily. Studies show that doing this before conception and during early pregnancy can reduce your baby's risk of neural tube defects by 70 percent.

Ginger and Turmeric

"Dried ginger is a more powerful anti-inflammatory agent than fresh," notes Dr. Weil. Capsules of dried, powdered ginger are sold in health food stores; some are standardized for content of active components. The recommended starting dose is 1 gram a day (usually two capsules) taken after a meal to avoid stomach irritation. "I know a number of people whose musculoskeletal and other ailments disappeared after using ginger in this way for several months. There is no reason not to stay on it indefinitely." Turmeric offers similar anti-inflammatory benefits, and some studies show the two may be even more powerful when paired. "I suggest you take a whole extract of turmeric, such as one prepared by the process of 'supercritical extraction,' which uses liquefied carbon dioxide as a solvent," Dr. Weil advises. "Turmeric may have a specific preventive effect against Alzheimer's disease. The population of rural India has one of the lowest rates of this disease in the world; daily consumption of turmeric may be a factor, because animal experiments with it demonstrate a protective effect. I believe it reduces the risk of cancer as well."

Grape Seed Extract

This is an excellent source of a group of flavonoids called proanthocyanidins, or PCOs. "Many practitioners recommend these supplements for the prevention and treatment of particular age-related diseases, including cardiovascular disease, cataracts, and macular degeneration. In the absence of specific ailments, they suggest a daily dose of 100 milligrams to maintain general health," advises Dr. Weil.

"You might consider these products for additional antioxidant support if you are not consuming enough dietary sources of flavonoids."

Grapefruit Seed Extract

I put ten drops of this in my water every day. It promotes healthy bacteria in the intestines and I think it helps balance your pH levels, so you stay alkaline, not acidic.

Milk Thistle

This herb has "an excellent reputation for protecting and enhancing liver function," says Dr. Weil, which makes it a powerful detoxifying agent. "Milk thistle is nontoxic and can be used for extended periods," he notes. "Anyone who drinks alcohol heavily, takes drugs or medications that can harm the liver, has abnormal liver function for any reason, works with solvents, or has a history of toxic exposures should take milk thistle. Look for extracts standardized to 70 to 80 percent silymarin, the active fraction, and take two capsules twice a day or as the label directs."

Saw Palmetto (For Men)

A growing number of studies suggest that saw palmetto can help men with benign, enlarged prostates, reports the CSPI.

Holistic Health Care

In addition to my daily regimen of vitamins and supplements, I rely on several different alternative therapies to maintain my health. Here's a quick primer to get you started in the world of holistic health care, with resources if you'd like to learn more. Remember that before beginning any alternative treatment, it is important to consult your doctor (or other health-care professional) and to find a reputable, trained, licensed practitioner.

- **Acupuncture.** This procedure, where a healer stimulates pressure points on your body with very thin needles (or sometimes her hands), originated in China more than two thousand years ago. It's used to treat everything from obesity to infertility, and studies have demonstrated that acupuncture can help osteoarthritis as well as soothe pain and nausea following dental operations and chemotherapy. Preliminary research also suggests that it can play a useful role in the treatment of headaches, back pain, carpal tunnel syndrome, asthma, menstrual cramps, fibromyalgia, addiction, and in stroke rehabilitation.

  To Learn More: Visit the American Academy of Medical Acupuncture at www.medicalacupuncture.org

- **Homeopathy.** This alternative medicine system is based on the theory that you can prevent or treat an illness by stimulating your body's defenses with very small doses of homeopathic remedies made from a wide array of herbs, essential oils, and floral essences. I swear by homeopathy and frequently use Young Living essential oils and Bach Flower Essences to stay healthy. I've found homeopathic remedies can work on simple complaints like indigestion and menstrual cramps and also on more serious issues, like keeping your hormones balanced, which is so important given the daily onslaught of hormone disrupting chemicals we face in our environment.

To Learn More: Visit the North American Society of Homeopaths at www.homeopathy.org; Bach Flower Essences are available at www.bachflower.com; Young Living essential oils are available at young living.us.

- **Massage Therapy.** There are more than eighty different kinds of massage therapies, ranging from Swedish to deep tissue to shiatsu, and which one you try is a matter of personal preference. They are all wonderful for reducing your stress level and maintaining your general sense of well-being. "Much of the information we need to heal is locked in our muscles and other body parts," writes Christiane Northrup, MD, in her book *Women's Bodies, Women's Wisdom: Creating Physical and Emotional Health and Healing.* "Getting a good massage will often release old energy blockages and help us cry or get rid of chronic pain from 'holding the world on our shoulders.'"

  To Learn More: Visit the American Massage Therapy Association at amtamassage.org.

- **Reiki.** This ancient Japanese practice is based on the belief that our bodies contain *ki,* or life-force energy fields. A Reiki master places his or her hands on or near your body in order to transmit *ki* and improve the flow and balance of your energy fields. Reiki is used to treat stress and chronic pain and improve your immune system and sense of mental well-being. At the Deirdre Imus Environmental Center for Pediatric Oncology, we also use Reiki to help patients recovering from surgery and chemotherapy. Some Reiki masters use crystals and other gemstones to neutralize negative energy; I keep pieces of malachite around my computer to protect me from the potentially dangerous electromagnetic fields it produces and sometimes carry aquamarine stones to give me more energy.

To Learn More: Visit the International Association of Reiki Professionals at www.iarp.org.

A Word about Exercise

If you really want to look and feel young and healthy, forget popping pills and try going for a walk. It has always been my personal belief that exercise truly is the root of good health. So often I meet women who think all they have to do is diet, diet, diet, and the truth is, you'll never get the body you want or improve your health if you don't exercise as well.

Let me first clarify that when I say "the body you want," I don't mean becoming super skinny. That's not healthy or sustainable! Being fit is about a lot more than a number on scale. Besides the physical benefits, you'll find that exercise also has the power to boost your immune system and improve your mental well-being.

So what kind of exercise should you be doing? Always consult a doctor first, because it will depend on your age and current fitness level. But the Centers for Disease Control recommends that all adults get a minimum of 30 minutes of moderate-intensity exercise (like walking) on most days, or 20 minutes of vigorous-intensity exercise (like running) on at least 3 days per week, as well as two days of strength training (involving 6 to 8 exercises, with 8 to 12 repetitions of each move).

Even with our increasingly busy lives, I think most of us can find 20 or 30 minutes a day to exercise—and once you start, you might find you want to do more! You should do anything that seems fun for you, whether that's walking, running, cycling, yoga, or Pilates—if you enjoy exercise, you'll find it much easier to stick with.

Further Reading

The world of holistic health care is far too enormous for me to do it justice here. If you are interested in learning more about the different forms of alternative medicine, I recommend the following titles. (All are available in bookstores or at www.amazon.com.)

- *Quantum Healing* by Deepak Chopra, MD

- *The Cure for All Cancers: Including over 100 Case Histories of Persons Cured* by Hulda R. Clark

- *Herbal Remedies for Women: Discover Nature's Wonderful Secrets Just for Women* by Amanda McQuade Crawford

- *Vibrational Medicine: The #1 Handbook of Subtle-Energy Therapies* by Richard Gerber, MD

- *Alternative Cures: The Most Effective Natural Home Remedies for 160 Health Problems* by Bill Gottlieb

- *Back to Eden* by Jethro Kloss

- The What Your Doctor May Not Tell You series by John R. Lee, MD

- *Enlivening the Chakra of the Heart: The Fundamental Spiritual Exercises of Rudolf Steiner* by Florin Lowndes

- *Women's Bodies, Women's Wisdom: Creating Physical and Emotional Health and Healing* and other titles by Christiane Northrup, MD (her Web site, drnorthrup.com, is another phenomenal resource)

- *A Woman's Guide to Male Menopause: Real Solutions for Helping Him Maintain Vitality and Virility* by Marc R. Rose, MD

- *The Natural Remedy Book for Women* by Diane Stein

- Wise Woman Herbal series by Susun S. Weed

- *Essential Oils Integrative Medical Guide: Building Immunity, Increasing Longevity, and Enhancing Mental Performance with Therapeutic-Grade Essential Oils* by D. Gary Young, MD

A Greener You

Herbal tea almost always does the trick and is soothing. For colds, I use eucalyptus oil in a bowl of hot water and inhale with a towel over my head. I also use zinc/echinacea/vitamin C lozenges and my colds don't last very long.

—Priya, 39, Dublin, Ohio

Chapter 10

Buy Green, Eat Green, Be Green

I hope by now you're feeling excited and hopeful about your new green life. By choosing to take these key steps to protect your own health, you've also committed to protecting the health of your family. I won't lie—the stakes are high because threats to our health and the environment continue to mount. And greening your life does require a bit of effort. You have to educate yourself about the world around you and ask questions every step of the way. But I think you'll agree that once you get started, it isn't as hard as it seems. It doesn't have to cost more, and it doesn't have to mean giving up comfort, style, or time.

In fact, greening your life isn't about sacrifice—it's about adding quality to your life, with a delicious and more nourishing diet that gives you the energy and vitality you need to get through your day, stave off disease, and maybe even lose a few pounds; with cleaner cosmetics and personal-care products that give you the glowing skin and shiny hair you've always wanted; with comfortable, beautiful clothes that are free of toxic dyes and are made by fairly paid workers who are treated with dignity; and with fewer drugs and more truly natural vitamins, minerals, and herbal supplements that keep you healthy without polluting our waters.

A cleaner, healthier lifestyle can bring us closer to nature and to the people we love. This is something I think we all crave—but our fast-paced lives and toxic environment don't always make it easy to have. As the need to do something about our environmental health crisis becomes more urgent, I predict that making green consumer choices will become an easier and more natural part of your daily life. Until corporate farmers and manufacturers clean up their act, however, we must remain vigilant and ask questions: What is a product's source? What ingredients does it contain and how well studied are they? What are the ramifications of its farming or manufacturing process? Is there a more sustainable, safer alternative I can buy?

Remember that building a greener world is a journey that we're all taking together. Share what you learn with your friends and family, to encourage them to join the Green Revolution too. Together we truly can make a difference. Here's to your health!

A Greener You Top Ten

Here is a checklist of the top ten things you can do today to make your life a little greener and cleaner. I encourage you to visit my Web site, dienviro .com, for more tips and to share your success stories.

1. Don't smoke, drink in moderation, and avoid secondhand smoke whenever possible—especially if you have children.
2. Exercise to improve your cardiovascular health, reduce your stress, sweat out toxins, and maintain a healthy weight.
3. Read food labels. Choose organic whenever you can and avoid foods that are grown with pesticides, hormones, and antibiotics.
4. Buy local. This supports your neighboring farmers and reduces energy consumption required by the global transport of goods.

Food from your farmers' market is healthier and fresher because it hasn't traveled thousands of miles to reach your dinner table.

5. Use the Skin Deep database (cosmeticsdatabase.com) to help you find cosmetics and personal-care products that are free of fragrance, parabens, and other toxic chemicals. Let companies know if they need a makeover. Ask them to sign the Compact for Safe Cosmetics, which is a pledge to substitute chemicals linked to birth defects, infertility, cancer, brain damage, and other serious health consequences with safer alternatives.

6. Go chlorine free on all your paper products (especially feminine hygiene needs) to reduce your exposure to dioxin, a carcinogen released when chlorinated products are incinerated.

7. Green your cleaning. Look for nontoxic alternatives like my Imus Greening the Cleaning products) to harmful household cleaners that contain bleach and other toxins. Baking soda, white vinegar, and lemon juice can handle a lot of your cleaning challenges. Visit imusranchfoods.com and dienviro.com for more information.

8. Reduce, reuse. Take care of the clothes you already have. Don't let a little wear send you on a shopping spree—swap with friends instead. When you do buy new, look for organic fabrics and nontoxic dyes manufactured in sweatshop-free conditions.

9. Explore alternatives to artificial estrogens. Women who have prolonged exposure to estrogens are at higher risk for breast cancer, and major studies continue to show an increased risk when postmenopausal women use hormone replacement therapy (HRT). Women who use both birth control pills

and—later in life—HRT face an even greater risk of breast cancer than those who use neither. Explore your options with your doctor.

10. Choose safer supplements. Check for the USP label and do your homework to make sure your supplements contain what they say they do and are free of contaminants.

Appendix 1

Favorite Vegan Recipes
from the Imus Ranch

Vegan cooking is not as difficult as people think. Here are a few of my best you'll-never-miss-the-meat recipes. For more ideas (whether you're feeding three or thirty), check out my cookbook, *The Imus Ranch: Cooking for Kids and Cowboys*. Remember: Choose organic ingredients whenever you can.

Mr. Martin's Maple-Glazed Pecans

Use these crunchy sweet pecans on salads, with desserts, or on stir-fried veggies. You can use the same recipe to make glazed walnuts as well.

Preparation Time: 3 minutes

2 cups raw pecans

½ cup maple syrup

¼ cup raw unrefined sugar

1 tablespoon sea salt

Preheat the oven to 350°F. Spread the pecans on a baking sheet and toast until lightly browned and fragrant, 8 to 10 minutes. Remove them from the oven and set aside. Heat the maple syrup and sugar in a medium saucepan over medium heat, stirring frequently, until boiling. Boil the mixture for 2 minutes, and then add the toasted pecans. Continue cooking, stirring to coat the pecans, about 30 seconds more. Spread the pecans onto a baking sheet to cool. Sprinkle with salt. Makes about 2½ cups.

Andy's Avocado Burger Melt

These delicious sandwiches make perfect weeknight meals. Store-bought veggie burgers come in so many brands and flavors—you can find a lot of variations and never feel as if you've eaten the same burger twice.

Preparation Time: 20 minutes
Cooking Time: 13 minutes

2 tablespoons olive oil

½ medium red onion, thinly sliced

4 vegetarian burgers

8 slices sourdough bread, toasted

2 to 4 tablespoons Dijon mustard

3 ounces soy Monterey Jack cheese, sliced

3 large plum tomatoes, thinly sliced

1 avocado, thinly sliced

Heat the oil in a large skillet over medium-high heat. When the oil is shimmering, add the onion and sauté until tender, about 5 minutes. Remove the onion from the pan, reduce the heat to medium low, and add the burgers. Cook, turning once, for 8 minutes, or until golden brown. Spread the toast with the mustard. Top four of the toast slices with burgers, then cheese, tomato, avocado, and sautéed onion. Top with the remaining slices of toast, cut in half, and serve warm. Makes 4 sandwiches.

Cold Three-Bean Salad

I like to make a big batch of this on the weekends to have on hand for quick, easy meals. It's great to pack in a glass Pyrex container and take to work for lunch, to spread on whole-grain crackers for a snack, or heated up inside a spelt tortilla for dinner.

Preparation Time: 45 minutes, plus overnight soaking
Hands on Time: 5 minutes

1 pound raw kidney beans

1 pound raw black beans

1 pound canned garbanzo beans (chickpeas), drained and
    rinsed

1 large red onion, diced

1 bunch parsley, finely chopped

2 to 3 cloves garlic, diced (or more, to taste)

¼ cup olive oil

⅛ cup balsamic vinegar

Sea salt, to taste

Soak the kidney and black beans overnight, then boil in a pot of water for 30 to 40 minutes until tender. Rinse them thoroughly under cold water, then mix with the chickpeas, red onion, parsley, and garlic. Toss with oil and vinegar, then season with sea salt to taste.

Kidney Bean Burritos

These are the epitome of healthy fast food—make a big batch, roll them up in non-chlorine-bleached wax paper, stick them in the fridge, and they'll be ready to grab and go.

> *Preparation Time:* 35 minutes, plus overnight
> *Hands on Time:* 5 minutes

1 pound raw red kidney beans

1 medium onion, diced

Diced garlic and parsley, to taste

6 soft spelt tortillas

1 cup salsa

Soak the kidney beans overnight, then boil them for 30 minutes, until tender. Drain and rinse. Mix with onion, garlic, and parsley, then use a fork to mash into a paste. Spread some paste on each tortilla and top with salsa, then roll. You can leave some of the beans unmashed, if you prefer a chewier texture.

Imus Ranch Guacamole

This guacamole is super easy to make. Instead of chopping up all the peppers, onions, and chiles used in most guacamole recipes, we begin with our own Imus Ranch Southwest Salsa. We love our salsa, but you can use any brand you prefer. To prevent darkening, squeeze some fresh lemon juice over the top of the guacamole before covering and refrigerating.

> *Preparation Time:* 8 minutes

4 ripe avocados, peeled and seeded

3 tablespoons fresh lemon or lime juice

4 cloves garlic, minced

½ cup salsa

1 tablespoon chopped cilantro

salt, to taste

Combine the avocados, juice, and garlic in a medium bowl; mash with the back of a fork or potato masher. Add the salsa, cilantro, and salt and mix well to blend flavors. Cover and transfer to refrigerator. Serve cold. Makes 4 cups.

Avocado, Raspberry, and Mango Salad

The smooth avocado, crunchy nuts, and sweet fruits in this salad offer a terrific combination of flavors and textures.

Preparation Time: 15 minutes

4 cups mesclun salad mix

2 cups spinach leaves

2 avocados, peeled and diced

¼ cup Imus Ranch Honey-Dijon Dressing (see below)

1 cup fresh raspberries

1 mango, peeled and diced

¼ cup Mr. Martin's Maple-Glazed Pecans (see page 235)

Combine the mesclun and spinach in a large bowl. Add the avocados and dressing and toss gently to combine. Transfer to a serving dish and top with the raspberries, mango, and walnuts. Serve with additional dressing on the side, if you like. Makes 4 servings.

Imus Ranch Honey-Dijon Dressing

We use sunflower or safflower oil in many of our dressings because they contain monounsaturated fat—which helps to keep the arteries supple and lubricated—as well as being high in linoleic acid, an essential fatty acid that is one of the major building blocks of the immune system.

Preparation Time: 5 minutes

¼ cup honey

⅓ cup balsamic vinegar

3 tablespoons Dijon mustard

1 organic egg or 2 tablespoons liquid egg substitute

½ cup olive oil

½ cup sunflower or safflower oil

1 tablespoon salt

½ teaspoon freshly ground black pepper

Combine the honey, vinegar, mustard, and egg in the container of a food processor and process 1 to 2 minutes. With the motor running, slowly add the oils through the feed tube until the dressing is thickened and well blended. If it seems too thick, add a small amount of water to thin it. Add salt and pepper. Makes 1½ cups.

Arlena Teitelbaum's Simple Smoothie

Arlena is our chef at the Imus Ranch and all the kids adore her delicious fruit smoothies. You can add strawberries, raspberries, or whatever other fresh, in-season fruit you have on hand.

Preparation Time: 5 minutes

1 organic ripe banana

¾ cup unsweetened organic soymilk

⅓ cup organic orange juice

Using a food processor or blender, pulse the banana until chopped. Add soymilk and pulse until the mixture starts becoming smooth. Add the orange juice and pulse until frothy. Serve immediately. Note: "Pulse" is a feature on many blenders, but simply turning a food processor on and off will produce similar results. Overblending the banana creates a heavier, thicker smoothie.

Basic Biscuits

Preparation Time: 10 minutes

1 cup organic unbleached flour

1 cup organic whole-grain flour (buckwheat, oat, spelt)

2 teaspoons aluminum-free baking powder

½ teaspoon sea salt

6 tablespoons organic coconut oil

¾ cup organic nut or soymilk

Preheat the oven to 400°F. Sift dry ingredients together. Incorporate the solid oil into the crumbled mixture, then add liquid to the dry

mixture and stir loosely. Do not overmix. Drop onto greased baking
sheets and bake 10 to 12 minutes. Serve warm.

For Bountiful Biscuits: Add any variety of dried fruits, nuts, or seeds.

Arlena's Balancing Breakfast Bars

These bars take a little longer to prepare, but they freeze well, and kids
love them.

Preparation Time: 25–30 minutes

2 ripe organic bananas

2 tablespoons organic cinnamon powder

1 teaspoon sea salt

1 cup organic agave nectar, divided

1¼ cup organic flaxseed, finely ground (flax meal), divided

⅓ cup purified water

1 cup organic sweet potato or pumpkin, mashed

2 cups organic carrots, shredded

2 organic apples, peeled and finely diced (or shredded)

3 cups organic rolled oats

1 cup organic oat flour

1 cup organic spelt flour

1½ cups organic almond butter

¾ cup organic coconut flakes

¾ cup organic walnuts (or pecans), finely chopped

Preheat oven to 350°F. Combine bananas, cinnamon, salt, ¾ cup
agave, 1 cup flax, and water until smooth. Add the sweet potato,

carrots, and apples. Add the oats and flours until fully incorporated. Grease a glass lasagna pan and bread pan. Place the mixture into the pans and spread/pat until evenly distributed (about ½ inch thick). Bake for 50 to 60 minutes. While the bars are baking, prepare the icing. Mix together the almond butter and remaining agave and flax until smooth. Cover and set aside. When the bars are cool, spread the almond mixture on top and then sprinkle with coconut and the nuts. Cut into small rectangles to serve.

Rio Grande Granola

We make this at the ranch and the kids all love its slightly chewy texture, fragrant spicy taste, and just the right amount of sweetness. Before baking, the mixture is somewhat sticky, so use a big wooden spoon to stir it. Store in an airtight container until you're ready to enjoy.

Preparation Time: 15 minutes

Cooking Time: 30–35 minutes

2 cups rolled oats

¼ cup raw unrefined sugar

¼ cup raisins

¼ cup toasted almonds

¼ cup sliced dehydrated banana (optional)

1 tablespoon ground cinnamon

⅛ teaspoon ground ginger

¼ cup safflower oil

1 to 2 tablespoons honey

½ teaspoon vanilla extract

Preheat the oven to 300°F. Combine the oats, sugar, raisins, almonds, banana (if using), cinnamon, and ginger in a large mixing bowl; stir until blended. In a separate bowl, stir together the oil, honey, and vanilla. Add the wet mixture to the dry mixture and stir with a wooden spoon until well blended. Then spread the mixture in a thin, even layer on a large baking sheet and bake 30 to 35 minutes, until lightly browned, stirring it twice and then patting down with a spatula. Scrape the granola onto a clean baking sheet and set aside to cool. Makes 6 ½-cup servings.

Arlena's Nourishing Truffles

Delicious for a snack when you're craving something sweet.

Preparation Time: 10 minutes, plus 15 minutes to roll truffles
Refrigeration Time: 1 hour

1 cup organic shredded coconut, divided

3 tablespoons local bee pollen (or toasted almonds coarsely
   ground)

8 tablespoons organic carob and/or cocoa powder

⅓ cup hot water

10 tablespoons organic almond butter

5 tablespoons organic brown rice syrup

3 tablespoons organic vanilla extract

2 tablespoons organic agave nectar

Combine ⅔ cup coconut and bee pollen (or almonds). Set aside. In a mixing bowl, combine carob and/or cocoa powder with hot water. Stir until completely dissolved. Add the other ingredients (including remaining ⅓ cup coconut). Mix thoroughly. Refrigerate mixture for an hour. Roll into 1-inch balls and set on a tray lined with unbleached wax paper. Dip each ball into the coconut mixture. Store finished truffles in the refrigerator and enjoy up to 7 days.

Arlena's Caramel Popcorn

Preparation Time: 12 minutes

3 tablespoons organic sunflower or canola oil

¾ cup organic popcorn

½ teaspoon sea salt

6 tablespoons melted Earth Balance natural spread

3 tablespoons organic evaporated cane juice

2 tablespoons organic blackstrap molasses

¼ cup organic agave nectar

Preheat oven to 225°F. Heat the sunflower oil and popcorn on medium high in a large stainless-steel pot with a tight-fitting lid. Move the pan around so the popcorn is coated with oil. Allow the corn kernels to begin popping. As they start to pop, turn the heat to medium and move the pan back and forth over the burner until all the kernels have popped. Next, pour the popcorn into a large stainless-steel or glass bowl and sprinkle with sea salt. Melt Earth Balance in the pan and whisk in the remaining ingredients. Pour the mixture over the popcorn, stirring the popcorn until it is evenly coated. Place coated popcorn evenly on two baking sheets lined with unbleached parchment paper. Bake on the middle oven rack for 15 minutes. Allow to cool and then transfer to a glass container.

Appendix 2

Buying Green: A Web Resource Guide

In addition to the Web sites I suggest for individual products throughout the book, these are excellent resources for finding more eco-friendly products at stores near you.

Food

- Local Harvest, a searchable map to farmer's markets and other local food sources: localharvest.org

- Eat Well Guide, a resource for sustainably and locally-raised food, especially humanely-raised animal products: eatwellguide.org

- United States Department of Agriculture's Agricultural Marketing Service guide to farmer's markets: ams.usda .gov/farmersmarkets

Cosmetics & Personal Care Products

- Environmental Working Group's Skin Deep Cosmetic Safety Database: cosmeticsdatabase.com

- Campaign for Safe Cosmetics: safecosmetics.org
- Teens for Safe Cosmetics: teensforsafecosmetics.org

Fashion

- One Percent For The Planet: onepercentfortheplanet .org
- Center for the New American Dream: newdream.org/ buy/

Health

- Public Citizen's Health Research Group: worstpills.org
- Consumers Union's Prescription For Change Campaign: PrescriptionForChange.org
- Consumer Reports' Best Buy Drugs: CRBestBuyDrugs .org

Vitamins & Supplements

- Consumer Lab, Inc: Consumerlab.com
- National Institutes of Health Office of Dietary Supplements: http:dietary-supplements.info.nih.gov
- Consumer Reports magazine: consumerreports.org
- Center for Science in the Public Interest: cspinet.org

Alternative Medicine

- American Academy of Medical Acupuncture: medical acupuncture.org

- North American Society of Homeopaths: homeopathy.org

- American Massage Therapy Association: amtamassage .org

- International Association of Reiki Professionals: iarp.org

Eco Shopping Lists

Food (Choose organic whenever possible!)

Organic Dairy

- Brown Cow Farm Yogurt (browncowfarm.com)

- Cowgirl Creamery Cheeses (cowgirlcreamery.com)

- Horizon Organic milk, yogurt, cheeses, cream cheese, butter, ice cream, sour cream and eggs (horizonorganic .com)

- Organic Valley Farms milk, soy milk, butter, sour cream, cheese, cottage cheese (organicvalley.coop)

- Stonyfield Farm yogurts, milk, and ice cream (stony fieldfarm.com)

Grass-Fed, Organic Beef:

- Applegate Farms (nitrite-free hot dogs and lunch meats, at applegatefarms.com)

- Grateful Harvest (albertsorganics.com)
- Niman Ranch (nimanranch.com)
- North Hollow Farm (vermontgrassfedbeef.com)

Certified Humane, Organic Pork:

- Applegate Farms (bacon, cured meats, ham)
- Caw Caw Creek Farm (heirloom pork, sausage, bratwurst, proscuitto, bacon, at cawcawcreek.com)
- Flying Pigs Farm (flyingpigsfarm.com)
- Niman Ranch

Certified Humane, Organic Poultry:

- Applegate Farms
- Alison's Family Farms (chicken, turkey, turkey bacon, at alisonsfamilyfarms.com)
- Murray's Chickens (murrayschicken.com)
- Wild Oats organic cage-free eggs (wildoats.com)

Safe to Eat Fish: (low mercury, not overfished or farmed destructively; ecofish.com is a great resource)

- Abalone (farmed)
- Anchovies
- Artic char (farmed)

- Barramundi (American farmed)
- Catfish (American farmed)
- Caviar (American or French farmed)
- Soft-shelled or steamer clams (farmed)
- Crab (trap-caught American Dungeness, Alaskan wild-caught imitation, Canadian snow, Floridian stone)
- Crawfish (American farmed)
- Croaker (Atlantic)
- Cuttlefish
- Herring
- Hoki
- Spiny or rock lobster (American, Australian, Baja west coast)
- Atlantic Mackerel (purse seine-caught)
- Mussels (American farmed)
- Oysters (Pacific farmed)
- Pollock (Alaskan wild-caught)
- Prawn (British Columbian wild-caught)
- Salmon (Alaskan wild-caught)
- Sardines
- Big-eye and mackerel scad (Hawaiian)
- Bay scallops (American farmed)
- Pink or wild-caught shrimp
- Longfin Squid (American, Atlantic)

- Striped bass (farmed)
- Sturgeon (farmed)
- Tilapia (American farmed)
- Rainbow Trout (American farmed)

Nuts and Seeds: (I buy from the bulk bins at my local health food store.)

- Raw pumpkin seeds (or tossed in safflower oil and sea salt, then baked for 20 minutes for a crunchy, tasty snack)
- Sunflower seeds
- Ground flax seeds
- Raw almonds
- Tamari almonds
- Raw filberts
- Raw cashews
- Raw walnuts
- Raw pecans

Fruits (Also found in bulk bins.)

- Dates
- Dried pineapple
- Dried banana chips
- Dried cherries
- Dried blueberries

Beans (Look for bulk bins or organic brands.)

- Black-eyed peas
- Green lentils
- Red lentils
- Black beans
- Kidney beans
- Pinto beans
- Navy beans
- Split peas
- Popcorn

Other Protein

- Tofu
- Tempeh

Milk

- Unsweetened Silk Soy Milk (silksoymilk.com)
- Strawberry and Banana VitaSoy Milk (vitasoy—usa.com)
- Carob Eden Soy Milk (edenfoods.com)

Extras for Cooking:

- Annie's Organic Yellow Mustard (annies.com)
- Annie's Organic Horseradish Mustard

- Apple cider vinegar

- Bionaturae Organic Extra Virgin Olive Oil (bionaturae .com)

- Bionaturae tomato paste

- Bionaturae crushed tomatoes

- Bionaturae strained tomatoes

- Cascadian Farms pickles (Cascadianfarms.com)

- Eden Organic Sauerkraut

- Creamy and whipped Earth Balance Butter (earth balance.net)

- Herbs: Fresh or dried organic basil, clove, fennel, garlic, parsley, turmeric

- Imus Ranch Salsa (imusranchfoods.com)

- Imus Ranch Balsamic Vinaigrette

- Mediterranean Organics Wild Capers (mediterrean organics.com)

- Muir Glen Organic Ketchup (muirglen.com)

- Muir Glen Fire-Roasted Tomatoes

- Natural Value Dijon Mustard (naturalvalue.com)

- Organic Tamari Soy Sauce

- Spectrum Organics Mayonnaise (spectrumorganics.com)

- Spectrum Organics Canola Oil

- Spectrum Organics Safflower Oil

Produce
Highest Pesticide Residue (always buy organic):

- Apples
- Bell and hot peppers
- Carrots
- Celery
- Cherries
- Grapes (imported)
- Green beans
- Nectarines
- Peaches
- Pears
- Potatoes
- Red raspberries
- Spinach
- Strawberries

Moderate Pesticide Residue (buy organic when you can):

- Apricots
- Blueberries
- Cantaloupe
- Grapes (domestic)
- Honeydew melons

- Oranges
- Collard greens
- Cucumbers
- Kale
- Lettuce
- Mushrooms
- Sweet potatoes
- Tomatoes
- Turnip greens
- Winter squash

Least Pesticide Residue (okay to buy conventional):

- Asparagus
- Avocados
- Apple juice
- Bananas
- Broccoli
- Cauliflower
- Cabbage
- Sweet Corn
- Kiwi
- Mangoes
- Orange juice

- Onions
- Papayas
- Pineapples
- Plums
- Sweet peas
- Tangerines
- Watermelon

Cooking Grains

- Barley
- Bulgur
- Millet
- Oats
- Quinoa
- Spelt

Breads

- Ezekiel 4:9 Organic Sprouted Flourless 100% Whole Grain Breads (foodforlife.com)
- Rudy's Organic Sourdough and Rosemary Olive Bread (Whole Foods and other health food stores)

Cereal

- Mochi organic sweet brown rice puffs (grainaissance .com)

Beverages

- Bionaturae Organic Nectars (Strawberry, Sicilian Lemon, and Wildberry, at bionaturae.com)
- Lakewood 100% Pure Organic Pineapple Juice (lakewoodjuices.com)
- R. W. Knudsen Just Black Cherry Juice and R. W. Knudsen Very Veggie Low Sodium Organic Juice (knudsenjuices.com)
- Herbal teas
- Filtered water

Frozen

- Cascadian Farms fruits and vegetables (cascadianfarms .com)
- Amy's Organic Pizza—I like their Rice Crust Spinach and Roasted Vegetable, which have non-dairy soy cheese (amys.com)

Whole Food Snacks

These healthy, delicious whole foods will satisfy your snack attacks without the junk.

- Organic Apples. Apples have crunch and a tangy flavor that's a good substitute for salty chips or pretzels. Or try bananas, apricots, kiwis, or any other fresh or dried fruits you enjoy.

- Plain Organic Yogurt. I prefer soy, but reduced-fat organic dairy is also a good option. Stir in a spoonful of ground flax for added nutrients.

- Edamame. Wyatt and I can eat these soybeans by the bowlful and they're so good for you!

- Olives and Tofu. Mix chunks of tofu (soy cheese works too) with a handful of black, red, or green olives. Also great with Edward and Sons' Brown Rice Crackers (edwardandsons.com).

- Almond Butter spread on a slice of Ezekiel 4:9 bread, topped with sliced bananas. strawberries, or peaches.

- DIY Granola. I mix organic dry rolled oats with walnuts, almonds, raisins, dried pineapples, blueberries, or cherries. You can experiment with the nuts, grains, and fruits you like to customize your own! Or see page 243 for my Rio Grande Granola.

- Tofu "Cheese" Salad. Cut up organic tofu mozzarella-style, in chunks, and combine with fresh tomatoes and Greek olives.

- Pita Breadsticks. Cut spelt bread pita into strips, brush them with olive oil, then sprinkle salt, pepper, and soy parmesan cheese on top. Bake on 350 degrees Fahrenheit for 10 minutes or until crispy and crunchy.

- Yellow Rice. Cook jasmine rice with lots of turmeric powder for a natural antioxidant meal.

Store-Bought Snacks

- Edward and Sons Brown Rice Snap Crackers (edwardandsons.com)

- Late July Classic Rich or Classic Saltine Crackers (latejuly.com)

- Mary's Gone Crackers (marysgonecrackers.com)

- New Morning Honey Graham Crackers (mannaharvest .net)

- NuGo Organic Bars (nugonutrition.com)

- Oskri Organics Sesame Seed Bars (oskri.com)

Once in a Blue Moon Favorites

- Root Beer Floats. Put two scoops of vanilla Soy Delicious ice cream in a parfait glass or tall drinking glass, then pour Virgil's Root Beer all over and serve with a straw.

- Hot Fudge Sundaes. I make these with organic Soy Delicious ice cream, Ah!laska's organic chocolate syrup, and soy whipped cream. Choose your favorite cut-up fruits for toppings. We love coconut, kiwi, strawberries, bananas, and raspberries.

- Sunspire Organic Chocolate (sunspire.com)
- Kettle Chips (kettlefoods.com)
- Fried Veggies. Roll sliced zucchini, leeks, eggplant, and tomatoes in a homemade batter of organic breadcrumbs, an egg, sea salt, pepper, and oregano (to taste) and fry in organic safflower or canola oil until brown and crispy.

Cosmetics & Personal Care Products

These are my favorite products. See Chapters 5 and 6 for more safe options.

Hair

- Avalon Organics Therapeutic Shampoo (avalonorganics .com)
- Aubrey Organics Natural Baby & Kids Shampoo
- Giovanni Positron Magnetic Energizing Shampoo (giovannicosmetics.com)
- John Masters Organics Shampoo (johnmastersorganics .com)
- Avalon Organics Hair, Bath, and Body Conditioner
- Dr. Hauschka Neem Hair Lotion (drhauschka.com)

Hair Dye

I highlight my blonde hair so I can avoid darker dyes, but there is just no good solution here—we need to pressure the hair industry to step up to the plate. John Masters Organics is a New York City salon that uses only ammonia-free herbal and clay based products.

Hair Styling

- Giovanni Electrix Magnetic Attraction Styling Gel and Gio Magnetic Force Styling Wax

- John Masters Organics Dry Hair Nourishment and Defrizzer

Bath

- Aubrey Organics Honeysuckle Soap Bar

- Pangea Organics soaps (pangeaorganics.com)

- Avalon Organic Liquid Soap

- Ortiz Mountain Full Moon Rose Petal Bath Soak, which is hand-made in small batches by Arlena Teitelbaum, our chef at the Imus Ranch (call 800.923.0072)

- Farmaesthetics Solar Sea Salt Rocks (farmaesthetics.com)

- SPA Technologies Sea Cal Bath Powder (spatechnologies .com)

Shaving Products

I never use depilatories or other chemical forms of hair removal. Instead I just shave with my organic shower gel or soap. If you have dry skin, try using an organic hair conditioner as shaving gel — it will moisturize your skin much better than most of the conventional products out there.

Oral Care

- Jason Organics Powersmile No Fluoride Toothpaste
- Dr. Young Living Dentarome toothpaste (youngliving.us)
- Dr. Young Living Kidscent Toothpaste
- Thieves ® Fresh Essence Plus Mouthwash (young living.us)

Deodorant

- Avalon Organics Roll-On Deodorant (Rosemary)
- Erbaviva Organic Deodorant (erbaviva.com)
- Sure Invisible Solid Antiperspirant & Deodorant, Unscented

Body

- Aubrey Organics Rosa Mosqueta Rose Hip Moisturizing Cream
- Dr. Hauschka Quince Body Moisturizer
- John Masters Organics Blood Orange and Vanilla Body Milk

- Susan Ciminelli Marine Lotion and Sensitive Skin Anti-Aging Cream (susanciminelli.com)
- Desert Essence Organics Coconut Hand and Body Lotion

Suncare

- Aubrey Organics Green Tea Sunblock for Children
- Aubrey Organics Saving Face Sunscreen Spray and Aubrey Organics Natural Sun SPF 25

Lips

- Dr. Hauschka Skin Care Lip Care Stick
- Dr. Hauschka Lipstick Novum
- Jane Iredale PureMoist Lip Colour in Babe
- Dr. Hauschka Novum Lip Gloss
- Alba TerraGloss (albabotanica.com)

Eyes

- Susan Ciminelli Eye Cream
- Kimberly Sayer of London Cellular Extract Eye Lift Gel (kimberlysayer.com)
- Dr. Hauschka Cleansing Milk

Eyeliner

- Jane Iredale Eye Pencil

Eye Shadow

- Jane Iredale PurePressed Eye Shadows
- Dr. Hauschka Eyeshadow Solo in Sunglow.

Mascara

- Jane Iredale PureLash Lengthening Mascara

Face

- Farmaesthetics Facial Cleanser with Lavender
- Tracie Martyn Purifying Cleanser (traciemartyn .com)
- Mychelle Blueberry Face Mask (mychelleusa.com)
- Susan Ciminelli Sea Clay Mask or Fresh Made Prune Mask
- Arlena Teitelbaum's Moroccan Red Clay and French Green Clay
- Arlena Teitelbaum's Ortiz Mountain Rose Water and Ortiz Mountain Lemongrass Spray
- Jane Iredale Pommisst (janeiredale.com)
- Kimberly Sayer of London Anti-Oxidant Daily Moisturizing Cream SPF 25 (kimberlysayer.com)

- Tracie Martyn Enzyme Exfoliant and Firming Serum
- SPA Technologies Oxygenated Renewal Complex

Concealer

- Jane Iredale Disappear Camouflage Cream

Foundation

- Jane Iredale Pressed Foundation
- Ecco Bella FlowerColor Natural Liquid Foundation

Blush

- Jane Iredale PurePressed Blush
- Dr. Hauschka Rouge Powder

Bronzer/Highlighting Powder

Dr. Hauschka Bronzing Powder and Translucent Bronze Concentrate (a liquid you can mix with your moisturizer or sunscreen).

Body Powder

- Farmaesthetics High Cotton Body Dust (I put it in my shoes and on my feet!)
- Cornstarch, arrow root, or baking soda from your kitchen are also highly effective

Insect Repellant

Put 30 to 50 drops of Dr. Young Living's Purification Essential Oil into a 16-ounce spray bottle filled with distilled water.

Fragrance/Perfume

I mix my own fragrance using Dr. Young Therapeutic Grade Essential Oils. Patchouli and clove are some of my favorite scents, but you should experiment to find the ones that work best with your own body chemistry.

Or try "i," the perfume created by Teens for Safe Cosmetics and the natural and organic personal care products company EO. It's made from organic jojoba oil, pure essential oils of blood orange, orange, jasmine, grapefruit, lime, sandalwood and vanilla (eoproducts.com).

Nail Products

I never use nail polish of any kind—instead I polish my nails by soaking them in hydrogen peroxide for two minutes once every week or two. This keeps them clean, shiny, and bacteria-free. If you do want polish, try Honeybee Gardens Water Colors Nail Enamel (Non Peel-Off) and their Odorless Nail Polish Remover (honeybeegardens.com).

Feminine Hygiene

Natracare Tampons and Pads (natracare.com)

Toilet Paper and Tissues

- 365 (Whole Foods)
- Ambiance
- April Soft
- Best Value
- Earth First
- Fiesta
- Fluff Out
- Green Forest
- Hankies
- Marcal
- Planet
- Pert
- Seventh Generation
- Softpac

Fashion

Couture:

- Armani (Armani.com)
- Anna Cohen (annacohen.com)
- Beyond Skin (beyondskin.co.uk)
- Camper (camper.com)

- Edun and Loomstate (loomstate.org)
- Linda Loudermilk (lindaloudermilk.com)
- Stewart + Brown (stewartbrown.com)
- Terra Plana (Terraplana.com)

Mid-Range:

- American Apparel (americanapparel.net)
- Eileen Fisher (eileenfisher.com)
- Levi's Organic Cotton (levis.com)
- Nau (nau.com)
- Patagonia (Patagonia.com)
- Tsonga Shoes (tsongausa.com)
- Ten Thousand Villages (tenthousandvillages.com)

Bargain

- Gap Organic Cotton (gap.com)
- H&M Organic Cotton (hm.com)
- Maggie's Functional Organic (organicclothes.com)
- No Sweat Apparel (nosweatapparel.com)
- Wal-Mart Organic Cotton (walmart.com)

Water

- Pūr Ultimate Slim Design Pitcher CR-800, purwaterfilter.com.

- Brita Faucet Filtration System OPFF-100, Brita.com

- Brita Aquaview Faucet Filtration System, Brita.com

- Pūr Ultimate Horizonal Faucet Mount FM-4900L, purwaterfilter.com

Supplements to Consider

See Chapter 9 for more details about what to look for when choosing vitamins and supplements.

- Multivitamin/Multi-mineral

- Alpha-lipoic acid (with or without acetyl-L-carnitine)

- Vitamin B_{12}

- Co-Q-10 (coenzyme Q or ubiquinone)

- Fish oil

- Folic acid (for women)

- Ginger

- Grape Seed Extract

- Grapefruit Seed Extract

- Milk Thistle

- Saw Palmetto (for men)

- Turmeric

Recommended Reading

Environment

Carson, Rachel. *Silent Spring.* Mariner Books (104th Edition). October 2002.

Davis, Devra Lee. *When Smoke Ran Like Water: Tales of Environmental Deception and the Battle Against Pollution.* Basic Books. January 2004.

Koss, Jethro. *Back to Eden.* Lotus Press. January 1997.

Pollan, Michael. *The Botany of Desire: A Plant's-Eye View of the World.* Random House. May 2002.

―――. *Second Nature: A Gardener's Education.* Grove Press. August 2003.

Schapiro, Mark. *Exposed: The Toxic Chemistry of Everyday Products and What's at State for American Power.* Chelsea Green Publishing. September 2007.

Eco-Friendly & Vegetarian Cooking

Barber, Dan and Joyce Goldstein. *Mediterrean Fresh: A Compendium of One-Plate Salad Meals and Mix-and-Match Dressings.* W. W. Norton. May 2008.

Bittman, Mark. *How to Cook Everything Vegetarian: Simple Meatless Recipes for Great Food.* Wiley. October 2007.

Katzen, Mollie. *The Vegetable Dishes I Can't Live Without.* Hyperion. October 2007.

Lappe, Anna and Bryant Terry. *Grub: Ideas for an Urban Organic Kitchen.* Tarcher. April 2006.

Madison, Deborah. *America: The Vegetarian Table.* Chronicle Books. September 1996.

————. *Local Flavor: Cooking and Eating from America's Farmers' Markets*. Broadway. June 2002.

————. *Vegetable Soups from Deborah Madison's Kitchen*. Broadway. February 2006.

————. *Vegetarian Cooking for Everyone*. Broadway (10th Anniversary Edition). November 2007.

————. *Vegetarian Suppers from Deborah Madison's Kitchen*. Broadway. November 2007.

Raven, Sarah and Dan Barber (Foreword). *In Season: Cooking with Vegetables and Fruits*. Universe. September 2008.

Waters, Alice. *The Art of Simple Food: Notes, Lessons, and Recipes from a Delicious Revolution*. Clarkson Potter. October 2007.

Food, Farming & Nutrition

Campbell, T. Colin and Thomas M. Campbbell II. *The China Study: The Most Comprehensive Study of Nutrition Ever Conducted and the Startling Implications for Diet, Weight Loss and Long-term Health*. Benbella Books. June 2006.

Epstein, Samuel S. *What's In Your Milk? An Expose of Industry and Government Cover-Up on the Dangers of the Genetically Engineered (rBGH) Milk You're Drinking*. Trafford Publishing. August 2006.

Imhoff, Daniel and Michael Pollan. *Food Fight: The Citizen's Guide to a Food and Farm Bill*. University of California Press. March 2007.

Jacobson, Michael F. *Six Arguments for a Greener Diet: How a Plant-Based Diet Could Save Your Health and the Environment*. Center for Science in the Public Interest. July 2006.

Lappe, Francis Moore. *Diet for a Small Planet*. Ballantine Books. August 1991.

Nestle, Marion. *Food Politics: How the Food Industry Influences Nutrition and Health*. University of California Press. October 2007.

————. *What to Eat.* North Point Press. April 2007.

Pollan, Michael. *In Defense of Food: An Eater's Manifesto.* The Penguin Press. January 2008.

————. *The Omnivore's Dilemma: A Natural History of Four Meals.* Penguin. August 2007.

Robbins, John. *Diet for a New America.* HJ Kramer. April 1998.

Robbins, John. *The Food Revolution: How Your Diet Can Help Save Your Life and Our World.* Conari Press. July 2001.

————. *Everything I Want to Do is Illegal: War Stories from the Local Food Front.* Polyface. September 2007.

Salatin, Joel. *Holy Cows and Hog Heaven: The Food Buyer's Guide to Farm Friendly Food.* Polyface. February 2005.

Singer, Peter. *Animal Liberation.* Harper Perennial. December 2001.

————. *In Defense of Animals: The Second Wave.* Wiley-Blackwell. September 2005.

Cosmetics & Personal Care

Ciminelli, Susan. *The Ciminelli Solution: A 7-Day Plan for Radiant Skin.* Collins. April 2006.

Malkan, Stacey. *Not Just a Pretty Face: The Ugly Side of the Beauty Industry.* New Society Publishers. November 2007.

Steinman, David and Samuel S. Epstein. *The Safe Shopper's Bible: A Consumer's Guide to Nontoxic Household Products, Cosmetics, and Food.* Wiley. July 1995.

Fashion

Chouinard, Yvon. *Let My People Go Surfing: The Education of a Reluctant Businessman.* The Penguin Press. October 2005.

Schor, Juliet B. *Born to Buy: The Commercialized Child and the New Consumer Culture.* Scribner. October 2005.

————. *The Overspent American: Why We Want What We Don't Need.* Harper Paperbacks. April 1999.

Healthcare & Medication

American Society of Health-System Pharmacists and the editors of Consumer Reports. *Consumer Drug Reference 2008.* Consumer Reports. January 2008.

Brownlee, Shannon. *Overtreated: Why Too Much Medicine is Making Us Sicker and Poorer.* Bloomsbury USA. September 2007.

Davis, Devra Lee. *The Secret History of the War on Cancer.* Basic Books. October 2007.

Wolfe, Sidney M., Larry D. Sasich, and Peter Lurie. *Worst Pills, Best Pills: A Consumer's Guide to Avoiding Drug-Induced Death or Illness.* Pocket. January 2005.

Vitamins & Alternative Healthcare

Chopra, Deepak. *Quantum Healing: Exploring the Frontiers of Mind/Body Medicine.* Bantam. 1990.

Clark, Hulda R. *The Cure for All Cancers: Including Over 100 Case Histories of Persons Cured.* New Century Press. June 1993.

Clement, Brian. *Vitamin Myth Exposed: Nature's Promise Betrayed.* Healthful Communications, Inc. April 2008.

Cooperman, Tod. *Consumerlab.com's Guide to Buying Vitamins & Supplements: What's really in the bottle?* Consumerlab.com. June 2003.

Epstein, Samuel S. and David Steinman and Suzanne Levert. *The Breast Cancer Prevention Program.* MacMillan. October 1998.

Gerber, Richard. *Vibrational Medicine: The #1 Handbook of Subtle-Energy Therapies.* Bear & Company. March 2001.

Gottlieb, Bill. *Alternative Cures: The Most Effective Natural Home Remedies for 160 Health Problems.* Rodale Books. October 2000.

Lee, John R. *What Your Doctor May Not Tell Your About: Breast Cancer: How Hormone Balance Can Save Your Life.* Grand Central Publishing. March 2005.

Lowndes, Florin. *Enlivening the Chakra of the Heart: The Fundamental Spiritual Exercises of Rudolf Steiner.* Rudolf Steiner Press. April 2000.

Mcquade Crawford, Amanda. *Herbal Remedies for Women: Discover Nature's Wonderful Secrets Just for Women.* Prima Lifestyles. April 1997.

Northrup, Christianne. *Women's Bodies, Women's Wisdom: Creating Physical and Emotional Health and Healing.* Bantam. October 2006.

Rose, Marc R. *A Woman's Guide to Male Menopause: Real Solutions for Helping Him Maintain Virility and Vitality.* Keats Publishing. March 2000.

Stein, Diane. *The Natural Remedy Book for Women.* Crossing Press. April 1992.

Weed, Susun S. *Wise Woman Herbal* series. Ash Tree Publishing.

Weil, Andrew. *Healthy Aging: A Lifelong Guide to Your Well-Being.* Anchor. January 2007.

Young, D. Gary. *Essential Oils Integrative Medical Guide: Building Immunity, Increasing Longevity, and Enhancing Mental Performance with Therapeutic-Grade Essential Oils.* Essential Science Publishing. April 2003.

Index

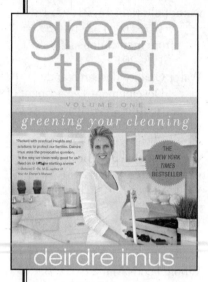

In *Greening Your Cleaning*, the first installment of the *New York Times* bestselling *Green This!* series, Deirdre Imus shows just how easy it is to make "living green" your way of life.

And don't miss the second volume in the series, *Growing Up Green!*, the parent-friendly, practical guide to raising a healthy child in our increasingly toxic environment.

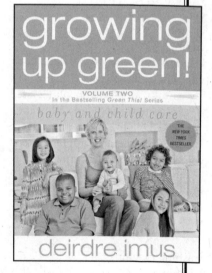